The Persecution and Trial
of *Gaston Naessens*

The Persecution and Trial of *Gaston Naessens*

The True Story
of the Efforts to Suppress
an Alternative Treatment for Cancer, AIDS,
and Other Immunologically Based Diseases

Christopher Bird

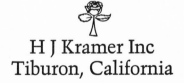

H J Kramer Inc
Tiburon, California

Published by H J Kramer Inc.
P.O. Box 1082
Tiburon, CA 94920

Editor: Nancy Grimley Carleton
Cover Design: Spectra Media
Book Production: Schuettge & Carleton
Composition: Classic Typography
Manufactured in the United States of America
10 9 8 7 6 5 4 3 2 1

Library of Congress Cataloging-in-Publication Data

Bird, Christopher, 1928–
    The persecution and trial of Gaston Naessans : the true story of
the efforts to suppress an alternative treatment for cancer, AIDS,
and other immunologically based diseases / Christopher Bird.
      p.   cm.
    Includes bibliographical references.
    ISBN 0–915811–30–8 (pbk.)
    1. Cancer—Alternative treatment. 2. Chronic diseases—
Alternative treatment. 3. Biological response modifiers—
Therapeutic use. 4. Naessens, Gaston—Trials, litigation, etc.
I. Title.
RC271.A62B57 1991
364.1'523'092—dc20
[B]   90–53451
                                 CIP

To Our Readers

The books we publish are our contribution to an emerging world based on cooperation rather than on competition, on affirmation of the human spirit rather than on self-doubt, and on the certainty that all humanity is connected. Our goal is to touch as many lives as possible with a message of hope for a better world.

Hal and Linda Kramer, Publishers

Contents

Foreword

Few individuals in their lifetimes have the privilege of so impacting established views that they are ridiculed, threatened, and vilified. Few individuals have the courage and intestinal fortitude to pursue truth as they know it in the face of withering attacks by those without vision—those who, even though they have eyes, do not see.

Fortunately for the world, there are a few rare mavericks like Gaston Naessens who understand the wisdom of the words of Orville Wright: "If we all worked on the assumption that what is accepted as true really is true, there would be little hope of advance."

Fortunately for the world, there exists Gaston Naessens, who exemplifies a perception of Felix Marti-Ibanez: "Great men, men who struggle alone for a great cause, are like great rivers. Debris may block their waters, but it never stops them from flowing."

This book is about a great river of human energy known by the name of Gaston Naessens—a name readers of this fascinating work by Christopher Bird will never forget.

Hugh Desaix Riordan, M.D.,
Director, Olive W. Garvey Center
for the Improvement of Human Functioning, Inc.,
Wichita, Kansas

Gratitudes

Many people have made the difficult task of writing this book under pressure an easier and more pleasant one than it would have been without their help.

First of all, I wish to thank Arthur Middleton Young, inventor of the Bell-47, the world's first commercially licensed helicopter, and founder of the Institute for the Study of Consciousness (Berkeley, California), and his wife, Ruth Forbes Young, founder of the International Peace Academy (New York), for their constant encouragement and moral support.

In Boston, Massachusetts, I gratefully acknowledge the logistical help and the "cheering section" provided by David Bird and Hannah Campbell of Bison Associates.

In Québec, I most appreciatively recognize: Christian De Laet, president of Development Alternatives–Canada (Montréal), for his cheerful concern, and for lending an erstwhile Californian an overcoat, scarf, and pair of warm mittens that allowed him to cope with the early onset of a chilly Québec winter; Ralph (Raoul) Ireland, operator of the Kebec Crystal Mines (Bonsecours), for all kinds of help proffered with joy and seasoned with humor; René Tongoc, president of Le Baron (Sherbrooke), and his agreeable hotel staff, for many courtesies that made ten weeks in a small "cell" seem less "imprisoning"; Jacques Gagné, proprietor of the Rock Forest Copying Service, for his gracious cooperation in this effort; and Brigitte Carbonneau (Sherbrooke), for her able and rapid transcription onto computer disk of day-to-day segments of a manuscript typed on the smallest of portable Olivetti typewriters.

Finally, my abiding thanks to Françoise and Gaston Naessens, for their good-humoredly taking time—when under extreme pressures of their own—to consult with me on the endless details that made this book possible.

Christopher Bird
Sherbrooke, Québec
February 1990

With the appearance of the American edition of this book, the author wishes additionally to thank retired Congressman Berkley Bedell, of Spirit Lake, Iowa; oil-and-gas "dowser" Dan Haley, of Forth Worth, Texas; and national radio-show hosts Dr. Robert Hieronimus and his wife Zohara, of Owings Mills, Maryland. All four have paid exemplary attention, and have provided exceptional assistance, to this effort.

In Mill Valley, California, Bruce L. Erickson merits many kudos for assiduously publicizing the truth about the "Naessens Affair" and, particularly, for his timely introduction to the current publishers.

And, in Atlanta, Georgia, none has grasped the great dimension of Naessens's contribution better than Shabari Red-Bird Cymerman, founder of that city's Gaia Institute, who has bent a strong oar to propel the vessel of its proclamation forward.

To Paul Sevigny, trustee and past president of the American Society of Dowsers (ASD), Danville, Vermont, I owe untold thanks for hours and hours of effort in mailing out the Canadian edition of this book from ASD's "Book and Supply" division, which he has so ably managed over a long period of time.

Especially appreciated is the devoted work of Nancy Grimley Carleton, Berkeley, California, who spent many editorial hours "combing and brushing" the text to free it from "lice and mites," and the vision of Hal and Linda Kramer, who, after an overnight reading of the Canadian edition, immediately decided they wanted to bring out this updated version for their wide American and world readership.

Christopher Bird
Bolinas, California
September 1990

Preface

*Most secrets of knowledge have been discovered by
plain and neglected men than by men of popular fame.
And this is so with good reason. For the men of popular
fame are busy on popular matters.*

Roger Bacon (c. 1220–1292),
English philosopher and scientist

This book is about a man who, in one lifetime, has been both
to heaven and to hell. In paradise, he was bestowed a gift
granted to few, one that has allowed him to see far beyond
our times and thus to make discoveries that may not properly
be recognized until well into the next century.

If a "seer's" ability is usually attributed to ephemeral "ex-
trasensory" perception, Gaston Naessens's "sixth" sense is a
microscope made of hardware that he invented while still
in his twenties. Able to manipulate light in a way still not
wholly accountable to physics and optics, this microscope
has allowed Naessens a unique view into a "microbeyond"
inaccessible to those using state-of-the-art instruments.

This lone explorer has thus made an exciting foray into
a microscopic world one might believe to be penetrable only
by a clairvoyant. In that world, Naessens has "clear seeingly"
descried microscopic forms far more minuscule than any
previously revealed. Christened *somatids* (tiny bodies), they
circulate, by the millions upon millions, in the blood of you,
me, and every other man, woman, and child, as well in that
of all animals, and even in the sap of plants upon which those
animals and human beings depend for their existence. These
ultramicroscopic, subcellular, living and reproducing forms
seem to constitute the very basis for life itself, the origin of

which has for long been one of the most puzzling conundrums in the annals of natural philosophy, today more sterilely called "science."

Gaston Naessens's trip to hell was a direct consequence of his having dared to wander into scientific terra incognita. For it is a sad fact that, these days, in the precincts ruled by the "arbiters of knowledge," disclosure of "unknown" things, instead of being welcomed with excitement, is often castigated as illusory, or tabooed as "fantasy." Nowhere are these taboos more stringent than in the field of the biomedical sciences and the multibillion dollar pharmaceutical industry with which it interacts.

In 1985, Gaston Naessens was indicted on several counts, the most serious of which carried a potential sentence of life imprisonment. His trial, which ran from 10 November to 1 December 1989, is reported in this book.

When I learned about Gaston Naessens's imprisonment, I left California, where I was living and working, to come to Québec and see what was happening. I owed a debt to the man who stood accused not so much for the crimes for which he was to be legally prosecuted as for what he had so brilliantly discovered during a research life covering forty years. To partially pay that debt, I wrote an article entitled "In Defense of Gaston Naessens," which appeared in the September-October issue of the *New Age Journal* (Boston, Massachusetts). That article has elicited dozens of telephone calls both to the magazine's editors and to Naessens himself.

Because the trial was to take place in a small French-speaking enclave in the vastness of the North American continent, I felt it important, as an American who had had the opportunity to master the French language, to cover the day-to-day proceedings of an event of great historical importance, which, because it took place in a linguistic islet, unfortunately did not made headlines in Canadian urban centers such as

Halifax, Toronto, Calgary, or Vancouver, not to speak of American cities.

When the trial was over, Gaston Naessens asked me, over lunch, whether, instead of writing the long book on his fascinating life and work that I was planning, I could quickly write a shorter one on the trial based on the copious notes I had taken. He felt it was of great importance that the public be informed of what had happened at the trial.

I agreed to take on the task because I knew that a great deal was at stake, not the least of which are the fates of patients suffering from the incurable degenerative diseases that Naessens's treatments, developed as a result of his microscopic observations, have been able to cure.

The tribulations and the multiple trials undergone by Naessens will come to an end only when an enlightened populace exerts the pressure needed to make the rulers of its health-care organizations see the light.

Part One
Setting the Stage

Chapter 1

Discovery of the World's Smallest Living Organism

When the great innovation appears, it will almost certainly be in a muddled, incomplete, and confusing form . . . for any speculation which does not at first glance look crazy, there is no hope.
Freeman Dyson, *Disturbing the Universe*

Early in the morning of 27 June 1989, a tall, bald French-born biologist of aristocratic mien walked into the Palais de Justice in Sherbrooke, Québec, to attend a hearing that was to set a date for his trial. On the front steps of the building were massed over one hundred demonstrators, who gave him an ovation as he passed by.

The demonstrators were carrying a small forest of laths onto which were glued, stapled, or thumbtacked placards and banners. The most eye-catchingly prominent among these signs read: "Freedom of Speech, Freedom of Medical Choice, Freedom in Canada!" "Long Live Real Medicine, Down With Medical Power!" "Cancer and AIDS Research in Shackles While a True Discoverer is Jailed!" "Thank you, Gaston, for having saved my life!" And, simplest of all: "Justice for Naessens!"

Late one afternoon, almost a month earlier, as he arrived home at his house and basement laboratory just outside the tiny hamlet of Rock Forest, Québec, Gaston Naessens had been disturbed to see a swarm of newsmen in his front yard. They had been alerted beforehand—possibly illegally—by officers of the *Sureté*, Québec's provincial police force, who promptly arrived to fulfill their mission.

As television cameras whirred and cameras flashed, Naessens was hustled into a police car and driven to a Sherbrooke jail, where, pending a preliminary court hearing, he was held for twenty-four hours in a tiny cell under conditions he would later describe as the "filthiest imaginable." Provided only with a cot begrimed with human excrement, the always elegantly dressed scientist told how his clothes were so foul smelling after his release on ten thousand dollars' bail that, when he returned home, his wife, Françoise, burned them to ashes.

It was to that same house that I had first come in 1978, on the recommendation of Eva Reich, M.D., daughter of the controversial psychiatrist-turned-biophysicist Wilhelm Reich, M.D. A couple of years prior to my visit with Eva, I had researched the amazing case of Royal Raymond Rife, an autodidact and genius living in San Diego, California, who had developed a "Universal Microscope" in the 1920s with which he was able to see, at magnifications surpassing 30,000-fold, never-before-seen microorganisms in living blood and tissue.*

Eva Reich, who had heard Naessens give a fascinating lecture in Toronto, told me I had another "Rife" to investigate. So I drove up through Vermont to a region just north of the Canadian-American border that is known, in French, as "L'Estrie," and, in English, as "The Eastern Townships." And, there, in the unlikeliest of outbacks, Gaston Naessens and his Québec-born wife, Françoise (a hospital laboratory technician and, for more than twenty-five years, her husband's only assistant), began opening my eyes to a world of research that bids fair to revolutionize the fields of microscopy, microbiology, immunology, clinical diagnosis, and medical treatment.

---

*"What Has Become of the Rife Microscope?," *New Age Journal*, (Boston, Massachusetts), 1976. This article has, ever since, been one of the *Journal*'s most requested reprints. It is reproduced in this book as Appendix A. Developments in microscopic techniques have only recently begun to match those elaborated by Naessens more than forty years ago

Let us have a brief look at Naessens's discoveries in these usually separated fields to see, step by step, the research trail over which, for the last forty years—half of them in France, the other half in Canada—he has traveled to interconnect them. In the 1950s, while still in the land of his birth, Naessens, who had never heard of Rife, invented a microscope, one of a kind, and the first one since the Californian's, capable of viewing living entities far smaller than can be seen in existing light microscopes.

In a letter of 6 September 1989, Rolf Wieland, senior microscopy expert for the world-known German optics firm Carl Zeiss, wrote from his company's Toronto office: "What I have seen is a remarkable advancement in light microscopy. . . . It seems to be an avenue that should be pursued for the betterment of science." And in another letter, dated 12 October 1989, Dr. Thomas G. Tornabene, director of the School for Applied Biology at the Georgia Institute of Technology (Georgia Tech), who made a special trip to Naessens's laboratory, where he inspected the microscope, wrote:

Naessens's ability to directly view fresh biological samples was indeed impressive . . . . Most exciting were the differences one could immediately observe between blood samples drawn from infected and noninfected patients, particularly AIDS patients. Naessens's microscope and expertise should be immensely valuable to many researchers.

It would seem that this feat alone should be worthy of an international prize in science to a man who can easily be called a twentieth-century "Galileo of the microscope."

With his exceptional instrument, Naessens next went on to discover in the blood of animals and humans—as well as in the saps of plants—a hitherto unknown, ultramicroscopic, subcellular, living and reproducing microscopic form,

which he christened a *somatid* (tiny body). This new particle, he found, could be cultured, that is, grown, outside the
bodies of its hosts (in vitro, "under glass," as the technical
term has it). And, strangely enough, this particle was seen
by Naessens to develop in a pleomorphic (form-changing)
cycle, the first three stages of which—somatid, spore, and
double spore—are perfectly normal in healthy organisms, in
fact crucial to their existence. (See Figure 1.)

Even stranger, over the years the somatids were revealed
to be virtually *indestructible!* They have resisted exposure to
carbonization temperatures of 200° C and more. They have
survived exposure to 50,000 rems of nuclear radiation, far
more than enough to kill any living thing. They have been
totally unaffected by any acid. Taken from centrifuge residues, they have been found impossible to cut with a diamond
knife, so unbelievably impervious to any such attempts is
their hardness.

The eerie implication is that the new minuscule life
forms revealed by Naessens's microscope are imperishable.
At the death of their hosts, such as ourselves, they return
to the earth, where they live on for thousands or millions,
perhaps billions, of years!

This conclusion—mind-boggling on the face of it—is not
one that sprang full-blown from Naessens's mind alone. A
few years ago, I came across a fascinating doctoral disserta-
tion, published as a book, authored by a pharmacist living
in France named Marie Nonclercq.

Several years in the writing, Nonclercq's thesis delved
into a long-lost chapter in the history of science that has all
but been forgotten for more than a century. This chapter concerned a violent controversy between, on the one side, the
illustrious Louis Pasteur, whose name, inscribed on the lin-
tels of research institutes all over the world, is known to all
schoolchildren, if only because of the pasteurized milk they
drink.

Figure 1: The Somatid Cycle

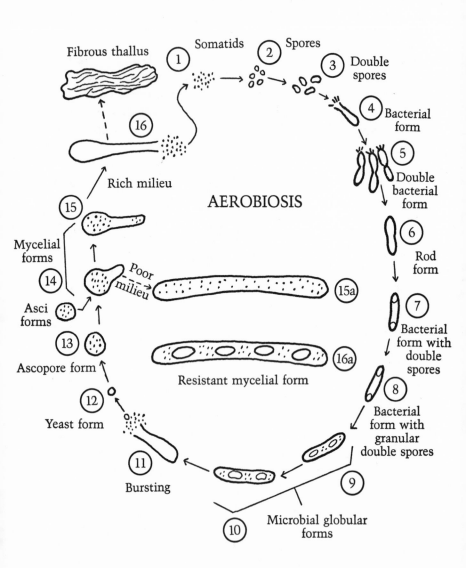

Credit: Courtesy of Gaston Naessens

On the other side was Pasteur's nineteenth-century contemporary and adversary, Antoine Béchamp, who first worked in Strasbourg as a professor of physics and toxicology at the Higher School of Pharmacy, later as professor of medical chemistry at the University of Montpellier, and, later still, as professor of biochemistry and dean of the faculty of medicine at the University of Lille, all in France.

While laboring on problems of fermentation, the breakdown of complex molecules into organic compounds via a "ferment"—one need only think of the curdling of milk by bacteria—Béchamp, at his microscope, far more primitive than Naessens's own instrument, seemed to be able to descry a host of tiny bodies in his fermenting solutions. Even before Béchamp's time, other researchers had observed, but passed off as unexplainable, what they called "scintillating corpuscles" or "molecular granulations." Béchamp, who was able to ascribe strong enzymatic (catalytic change-causing) reactions to them, was led to coin a new word to describe them: *microzymas* (tiny ferments).

Among these ferments' many peculiar characteristics was one showing that, whereas they did not exist in *chemically pure* calcium carbonate made in a laboratory under artificial conditions, they were abundantly present in *natural* calcium carbonate, commonly known as *chalk*. For this reason, the latter could, for instance, easily "invert" cane sugar solutions, while the former could not.

With the collaboration of his son, Joseph, and Alfred Estor, a Montpellier physician and surgeon, Béchamp went on to study microzymas located in the bodies of animals and came to the startling conclusion that the tiny forms were far more basic to life than cells, long considered to be the basic building blocks of all living matter. Béchamp thought them to be fundamental elements responsible for the activity of cells, tissues, organs, and indeed whole living organisms, from bacteria to whales, and larks to human beings. He even found them present in life-engendering eggs, where they were responsible for the eggs' further development while themselves undergoing significant changes.

So, nearly a century before Gaston Naessens christened his somatid, his countryman, Béchamp, had come across organisms that, as Naessens immediately recognized, seem to be "cousins," however many times removed, of his own "tiny bodies."

Most incredible to Béchamp was the fact that, when an event serious enough to affect the whole of an organism occurred, the microzymas within it began working to disintegrate it totally, while at the same time continuing to survive. As proof of such survival, Béchamp found these microzymas in soil, swamps, chimney soot, street dust, even in air and water. These basic and apparently eternal elements of which we and all our animal relatives are composed survive the remnants of living cells in our bodies that disappear at our death.

So seemingly indestructible were the microzymas that Béchamp could even find them in limestone dating to the Tertiary, the first part of the Cenozoic Era, a period going back sixty million years, during which mammals began to make their appearance on earth.

And it could be that they are older still, far older. Professor Edouard Boureau, a French paleontologist, writes in his book *Terre: Mère de la Vie* (Earth: Mother of Life), concerning problems of evolution, that he had studied thin sections of rock, over three billion years old, taken from the heart of the Sahara Desert. These sections contained tiny round coccoid forms, which Boureau placed at the base of the whole of the evolutionary chain, a chain that he considers might possibly have developed in one of three alternative ways. What these tiny coccoid forms could possibly be, Boureau does not actually know, but, from long study, he is sure about the fact they were around that long ago.

When I brought the book to Naessens's attention, he told

me, ingenuously and forthrightly: "I'd sure like to have a few samples of moon rocks to section and examine at my microscope. Who knows, we might find somatid forms in them, the same traces of primitive life that exist on earth!"

Over years of careful microscopic observation and laboratory experimentation, Naessens went on to discover that if and when the immune system of an animal or human being becomes weakened or destabilized, the normal three-stage cycle of the somatid goes through thirteen more successive growth stages to make up a total of *sixteen* separate forms, each evolving into the next. (See diagram of the somatid cycle on page 6).

All of these forms have been revealed clearly and in detail by motion pictures, and by stop-frame still photography, at Naessens's microscope. Naessens attributes this weakening, as did Béchamp, to *trauma*, brought on by a host of reasons, ranging from exposure to various forms of radiation or chemical pollution to accidents, shocks, depressed psychological states, and many more.

By studying the somatid cycle as revealed in the blood of human beings suffering from various degenerative diseases such as rheumatoid arthritis, multiple sclerosis, lupus, cancer, and, most recently, AIDS, Naessens has been able to associate the development of the forms in the sixteen-stage pathological cycle with all of these diseases. A videocassette showing these new microbiological phenomena is available. Among other things, it shows that when blood is washed to remove all somatids *external* to the blood's red cells, then heated, somatids latently present in a liquid state *within* the red blood cells themselves take concrete form and go on to develop into the sixteen-stage cycle. "This," says Naessens, "is what happens when there is immune system disequilibrium." It is not yet known exactly how or why or from what the somatids take shape. Of the some 140 proteins in red blood cells, many may play a role in the process. The appearance of somatids inside red blood cells is thus an enigma as puzzling as the origin of life itself. I once asked Naessens, "If there were no somatids, would there be no life?" "That's what I believe," he replied.

Even more importantly, Naessens has been able to predict the eventual onset of such diseases long before any clinical signs of them have put in an appearance. In other words, he can "prediagnose" them. And he has come to demonstrate that such afflictions have a common functional principle, or basis, and therefore must not be considered as separate, unrelated phenomena as they have for so long been considered in orthodox medical circles.

Having established the somatid cycle in all its fullness, Naessens was able, in a parallel series of brilliant research steps, to develop a treatment for strengthening the immune system. The product he developed is derived from camphor, a natural substance produced by an East Asian tree of the same name. Unlike many medicinals, it is injected into the body, not intramuscularly or intravenously, but *intralymphatically*—into the lymph system, via a lymph node, or ganglion, in the groin.

In fact, one of the main reasons the medical fraternity holds the whole of Naessens's approach to be bogus is its assertion that intralymphatic injection is impossible! Yet the fact remains that such injection is not only possible, but simple, for most people to accomplish, once they are properly instructed in how to find the node. While most doctors are never taught this technique in medical school, it is so easy that laypeople have been taught to inject, and even to self-inject, the camphor-derived product within a few hours.

The camphor-derived product is named "714-X"—the 7 and the 14 refer to the seventh letter "G" and the fourteenth letter "N" of the alphabet, the first letters of the inventor's first and last names, and the X refers to the twenty-fourth letter of the alphabet, which denotes the year of Naessens's birth, 1924. When skillfully injected, 714-X has, in over seventy-five percent of cases, restabilized, strengthened, or otherwise enhanced the powers of the immune system, which then goes about its normal business of ridding the body of disease.

Let us for a moment return to the work and revelations of Antoine Béchamp. As already noted, with the fairly primitive microscopic technology available in Béchamp's day, it was almost incredible that he was seemingly able to make microbiological discoveries closely paralleling, if not completely matching, those of Naessens nearly a hundred years later. We have already alluded to the fact that the microzymas in traumatized animals did not remain passive, as before, but, on the contrary, became highly active and began to destroy the bodies of their hosts, converting themselves to bacteria and other microbes in order to carry out that function.

While the terminology is not exactly one that Gaston Naessens would use today, the principles of trauma and of destruction of the body are shared in common by the two researchers. Had Béchamp had access to Naessens's microscope, he, too, might have established the somatid cycle in all the detail worked out by Naessens.

So what happened to Béchamp and his twentieth-century discoveries made in the middle of the nineteenth century? The sad fact is that, because he was modest and retiring— just like Gaston Naessens—his work was overshadowed by that of his rival. All of Pasteur's biographies make clear that he was, above all, a master of the art of self-promotion. But, odd as it seems, the same biographies do not reveal any hint of his battle with Béchamp, many of whose findings Pasteur, in fact, plagiarized.

Even more significant is that while Béchamp, as we have seen, championed the idea that the cause of disease lay *within* the body, Pasteur, by enouncing his famous "germ theory," held that the cause came from *without*. In those days, little was known about the functioning of the immune system, but what else can explain, for instance, why some people survived the Black Plague of the Middle Ages, while countless others died like flies? And one may add that Royal Raymond Rife's microscope, like that of Naessens, allowed him to state unequivocally that "germs are not the *cause* but the *result* of disease!" Naessens independently adopted this view as a result of his biological detective work. The opposite view, which won the day in Pasteur's time, has dominated medical philosophy for over a century, and what amounted to the creation of a whole new worldview in the life sciences is still regarded as heretical!

Yet the plain fact is that, based on Naessens's medical philosophy as foreshadowed by Béchamp and Rife, up to the present time, Naessens's treatment has arrested and reversed the progress of disease in over one thousand cases of cancer (many of them considered terminal), as well as in several dozen cases of AIDS, a disease for which the world medical community sadly states that it has as yet no solution whatsoever. Suffering patients of each sex, and of ages ranging from the teens to beyond the seventies, have been returned to an optimal feeling of well-being and health.

A layperson having no idea of the scope of Naessens's discoveries, or their full meaning and basic implications, might best be introduced to them through Naessens's explanation to a visiting journalist. "You see," began Naessens, "I've been able to establish a life cycle of forms in the blood that add up to no less than a brand new understanding for the *very basis of life*. What we're talking about is an *entirely new biology*, one out of which has fortunately sprung practical applications of benefit to sick people, even before all of its many theoretical aspects have been sorted out." At this point, Naessens threw in a statement that would startle any biologist, particularly a geneticist: "The somatids, one can say, are *precursors* of DNA. Which means that they somehow supply a 'missing link' to an understanding of that remarkable molecule that up to now has been considered as an all but irreducible building block in the life process."*

If somatids were a "missing link" between the living and the nonliving, then what, I wondered aloud in one of my meetings with Françoise Naessens, would be the difference between them and viruses, a long debate about the animate or inanimate nature of which has been going on for years? There was something, was there not, about the somatid that related to its nonreliance and nondependence upon any surrounding milieu needed by the virus, if it were to thrive.

"Yes," agreed Françoise, "to continue its existence, the virus needs a supportive milieu, say, an artificially created

---

*Intriguing is a recent discovery by Norwegian microbiologists. On 10 August 1989, as Naessens was preparing for trial, the world's most prestigious scientific journal, *Nature* (United Kingdom), ran an article entitled "High Abundance of Viruses Found in Aquatic Environments." Authored by Ovind Bergh and colleagues at the University of Bergen, it revealed that, for the first time, in natural unpolluted waters, hitherto considered to have extremely low concentrations of viruses, there exist up to 2.5 trillion strange viral particles for each liter of liquid. Measuring less than 0.2 microns, their size equates to the largest of Naessens's somatids. Much too small for any larger marine organism to ingest, the tiny organisms are upsetting existing theories on how pelagic life systems operate.

In light of Gaston Naessens's theory that his somatids are DNA precursors, it is fascinating that the Norwegian researchers believe that the hordes upon hordes of viruses might account for DNA's being inexplicably dissoved in seawater. Another amazing implication of the high viral abundance is that routine viral infection of aquatic bacteria could be explained by a significant exchange of genetic material. As Evelyn B. Sherr, of the University of Georgia's Marine Institute on Sapelo Island, writes in a sidebar article in the same issue of *Nature:* "Natural genetic engineering experiments may have been occurring in bacterial populations, perhaps for eons." What connection the aqua-viruses may have with Naessens's somatids is a question that may become answerable when Naessens has the opportunity to observe them at his microscope and compare them with the ones he has already found in vegetal saps and mammalian blood.

test-tube culture, or something natural, like an egg. If the virus needs this kind of support for growth, either in vivo or in vitro, a 'helping hand,' as it were, the somatid is able to live autonomously, either in a 'living body,' or 'glass-enclosed.' This has something to do with the fact that, while the virus is a *particle* of DNA, a piece of it, the somatid is, as we've already said, a 'precursor' of DNA, something that leads to its creation."

To try to get to the bottom of this seemingly revolutionary pronouncement, I later asked Françoise to set down on paper some further exposition of it. She wrote:

We have come to the conclusion that the somatid is no less than what could be termed a *concretization of energy.* One could say that this particle, one that is "initially differentiated," or materialized in the life process, possesses genetic properties transmissible to living organisms, animal or vegetal. Underlying that conclusion is our finding that, in the *absence* of the normal three-stage cycle, *no cellular division can occur!* Why not? Because it is the normal cycle that produces a special growth hormone that permits such division. We believe that hormone to be closely related, if not identical, to the one discovered years ago by the French Nobel Laureate Alexis Carrel, who called it a *trephone.*

The best experimental proof backing up this astounding disclosure, Françoise went on, begins with a cube of fresh meat no different from those impaled on shish kebab skewers. After being injected with somatids taken from an in vitro culture, the meat cube is placed in a sealed vessel in which a vacuum is created. With the cube now protected from any contamination from the ambient atmosphere, and anything that atmosphere might contain that could act to putrefy the meat, the vessel is subsequently exposed during the day to natural light by setting it, for instance, next to a window.

Harboring the living, indestructible somatids as it does, the meat cube in the vessel will, thenceforth, not rot, as it surely would have rotted had it not received the injection. Retaining its healthy-looking color, it not only remains as fresh as when inserted into the vessel, but progressively increases in size, that is, it continues to grow, just as if it were part of a living organism.

Could a meat cube, animated by somatids, if somehow also electrically stimulated, keep on growing to revive the steer or hog from which it had been cut out? The thought flashed inanely through my mind. Maybe there *was* something electrical about the somatid? Before I could ask that question of her, Françoise seemed to have already anticipated it.

"The 'tiny bodies' discovered by Naessens," she went on, "are fundamentally electrical in nature. In a liquid milieu, such as blood plasma, one can observe their electrical charge and its effects. For the *nuclei* of these particles are *positively* charged, while the *membranes*, coating their exteriors, are *negatively* charged. Thus, when they come near one another, they are automatically mutually repulsed just as if they were the negative poles of two bar magnets that resist any manual attempt to hold them together."

"Well," I asked, "isn't that the same as for cells, whose nuclei and membranes are, respectively, considered to have plus, and minus, electrical charges?"

"Certainly," she replied, "with the difference that, in the case of the somatids, the energetic release is very much larger. Somatids are actually tiny living condensers of energy, the smallest ever found."

I was thunderstruck. What, I mused, would the great Hungarian scientist Albert Szent-Györgyi, winner of the Nobel prize for his discovery of ascorbic acid (vitamin C) and many other awards, have had to say had he, before his recent death, been aware of Naessens's discoveries? For it was Szent-Györgyi who, abandoning early attempts to get at the "secret of life" at the level of the molecule, had predicted, prior to World War II, when still living and working in Hungary, that such a secret would eventually be discovered at the level of the electron, or other electrically related atomic particles!*

Probing further into the world of the somatid and its link to life's basis and hereditary characteristics, I asked Françoise if Naessens had done any experiments to show how somatids might produce genetic effects on living organisms.

"I'll tell you, now, about one experiment we have repeated many times," she answered, "whose results are hard for any orthodox biologist to swallow. Before describing it, let me add that it is our belief—as it was also Antoine Béchamp's—that each of our bodily organs possesses somatids of varying, as yet indescribable, natures that are specific to it alone. But the whole ensemble, the 'family' of these varying forms, collectively circulates, either in the circulatory or the lymph system. On the basis of this experiment, we hold that, as a group, they contain the hereditary characteristics of each and every individual being."

As described by Françoise, the experiment begins by extracting somatids from the blood of a rabbit with white fur. A solution containing them is then injected, at a dose of one cubic centimeter per day, into the bloodstream of a rabbit with black fur, for a period of two weeks running. Within approximately one month, the fur of the black rabbit begins to turn a grayish color, half of the hairs of which it is composed having turned white. In a reverse process, the fur of a white rabbit, injected with somatids from a black one, also begins to turn gray.

*For more recent discoveries relating to the electrical basis for life, readers are also referred to two fascinating books by Dr. Robert O. Becker, *The Body Electric* (New York: Quill, William Morrow, 1985) and *Cross Currents* (Los Angeles: J. P. Tarcher, 1990).

Astonishing as this result, with its "genetic engineering" implications, might be, the effect of such "somatid transfer" from one organism to another also, said Françoise, produces another result offering great insight into the role played by the somatid in the immunological system. "When a patch of skin," she continued, "is cut from the white rabbit and grafted onto the empty space left after cutting a patch of similar size from the black rabbit, the graft shows *none of the signs of rejection* that normally take place in the absence of somatid transfer." What this might bode for the whole technique of organ transplant, attempts at which have been bedeviled by the "rejection syndrome," we shall let readers—especially medically trained readers—ponder.

Chapter 2
Gaston Naessens's Life and Work

Is it not living in a continual mistake to look upon diseases, as we do now, as separate entities, which must exist, like cats and dogs, instead of looking at them as conditions, like a dirty and a clean condition, and just as much under our control; or rather as the reactions of a kindly nature, against the conditions in which we have placed ourselves?

Florence Nightingale, 1860 (seventeen years before Pasteur announced his germ theory), cited in *Pasteur: The Germ Theory Exploded* by R. B. Pearson

Even a single discovery as striking as those made by Naessens in the five interlinked areas detailed in the previous chapter could, by itself, justifiably be held remarkable. That Naessens was able to make all five discoveries, each in what can be termed its own discipline, might seem to be a feat taken from the annals of science fiction.

And that is exactly the point of view adopted by the medical authorities of the province of Québec. Worse still, those same authorities have branded Naessens an out-and-out charlatan, calling his camphor-derived 714-X product fraudulent and the whole of his theory about the origin of degenerative disease and the practice of its treatment, not to add the rest of his "New biology," no more than "quackery."

Spearheading the attack was Augustin Roy, a doctor of medicine, but one who—like Morris Fishbein, M.D., for many years "Tsar" of the American Medical Association—actually practiced medicine for only a brief period of his life.

18

How did a researcher such as Gaston Naessens, endowed with genius, come to land in so dire a situation? Let us briefly review some of the story of his life and work, about which, during repeated trips to Rock Forest from the United States, I came to learn more and more.

Gaston Naessens was born on 16 March 1924, in Roubaix, in northern France, near the provincial capital of Lille, the youngest child of a banker who died when his son was only eleven years old. In very early childhood, Gaston was already showing precocity as an inventor. At the age of five, he built a little moving automobile-type vehicle out of a "Mechano" set and powered it with a spring from an old alarm clock.

Continuing to exhibit unusual manual dexterity, a few years later Gaston constructed his own home-built motorcycle, then went on to fashion a miniairplane large enough to carry him aloft. It never flew, for his mother, worried he would come to grief, secretly burned it on the eve of its destined takeoff.

After graduation from the Collège Universitaire de Marc-en Baroeul, a leading prep school, Gaston began an intensive course in physics, chemistry, and biology at the University of Lille. When France was attacked and occupied by Nazi forces during World War II, young Gaston, together with other fellow students, was evacuated to southern France, where, in exile near Nice, he had the highly unusual opportunity to receive the equivalent of a full university education at the hands of professors also displaced from Lille.

By the war's end, Gaston had been awarded a rare diploma from the Union Nationale Scientifique Française, the quasi-official institution under whose roof the displaced students pursued their intensive curriculum. Unfortunately, in an oversight that has cost him dearly over the years, Naessens did not bother to seek an "equivalence" from the new republican government set up by General Charles de Gaulle. He thus, ever since, has been accused of never having received an academic diploma of any kind.

Inspired by his teachers, and of singular innovative bent, Gaston, eschewing further formal education—"bagage universitaire" as he calls it—set forth on his own to develop his microscope and begin his research into the nature of disease. In this determination, he was blessed by having what in French is called a *jeunesse dorée*, a gilded childhood—"born with a silver spoon in his mouth," as the English equivalent has it. His mother afforded him all that was needed to equip his own postwar laboratory at the parental home.

His disillusion in working in an ordinary laboratory for blood analysis spurred Gaston into deciding to go free-lance as a researcher. Even his mother was worried about Gaston's unorthodox leanings. She clearly understood that her son was unhappy with all he had read and been taught. As he was to put it: "She told me what any mother would tell her son: 'It's not you who will make any earth-shaking discoveries, for there have been many, many researchers working along the same lines for decades.' But she never discouraged me, never prevented me from following my own course, and she helped me generously, financially speaking."

Gaston Naessens knew that there was something in the blood that eluded definition. It had been described in the literature as *crasse sanguine* (dross in the blood), and Naessens had been able to descry it, if only in a blurry way, in the microscopic instruments up to then available to him. What was needed was a brand new microscope, one that could see "farther." He thought he knew how to build one and, at twenty-one, he determined to set about doing so.

In the design of the instrument that would open a vista onto a new biological world, Naessens was able to enjoin the technical assistance of German artisans in the village of Wetzlar, in Germany, where the well-known German optical company Leitz had been located before the war. The artisans were particularly helpful in checking Naessens's original ideas on the arrangement of lenses and mirrors. The electronic manip-

ulation of the light source itself, however, was entirely of
Gaston's own private devising. When all aspects of the problem seemed to have been solved, Naessens was able to get the
body of his new instrument constructed by Barbier-Bernard
et Turenne, technical specialists and military contractors
near Paris.

Readers may fairly ask why Naessens's "Twenty-first–
century" instrument, which has been called a "somatoscope"
due to its ability to reveal the somatid, has never been patented
and manufactured for wide use. To understand the difficulty,
we should "fast forward" to 1964, the year Naessens arrived
in Canada. Hardly having found his footing on Canadian soil,
he received a handwritten letter, dated 3 May, from one of
the province's most distinguished physicists, Antoine Aumont,
who worked in the Division for Industrial Hygiene of the
Québec Ministry of Health.

Aumont, who had read about Naessens's special microscope in the press, had taken the initiative of visiting Naessens in his small apartment in Duvernay, near Montréal, to
see, and see through, the instrument with his own eyes. Aumont wrote:

Many thanks for having accorded me an interview that impressed me far more than I can possibly
describe.

I have explained to you why my personal opinions
must not be considered as official declarations. But, after thinking over all that you showed, and told me, during
my recent visit, I have come to unequivocal conclusions
on the physical value of the instrumentation you are using to pursue your research.

As I told you, if my knowledge of physics and mathe-
matics can be of service to you, I would be very glad to
put them at your disposition.

It can be deduced that Aumont's enthusiasm for what he had seen caused a stir in the Québec Ministry of Health, for, on 17 July, Naessens received an official letter from that office stating that the minister was eager to have his microscope "officially examined" if its inventor would "furnish in writing details concerning this apparatus, including all its optical, and other, particularities, as well as its powers of magnification, so that experts to be named by the minister can evaluate its unique properties."

In reply to this letter, Naessens's lawyer sent a list of details as requested and stated: "You will, of course, understand that it is impossible for Monsieur Naessens to furnish you, in correspondence, the complete description of a highly novel microscope which is, moreover, unprotected by any patent." Then, to explain why no patent had yet been granted, he added a key phrase: "since its *mathematical constants have, up to the present, not been elucidated in spite of a great deal of tiresome work performed in that regard.*" In other words, it seemed that Aumont and his colleagues had been unable to explain the superiority of the microscope in terms of all the known laws of optics and it still seems that, so far, no one else has been able to do so.

There have been interesting recent reports on new microscopes being developed that apparently rival the magnification powers of Naessens's somatoscope. It would seem, however, that the 150 angstroms of resolution achieved by Naessens's instrument has not yet been matched.

The Los Angeles–based World Research Foundation's flyer, presenting its autumn (1990) conference "New Directions for Medicine . . . Focusing on Solutions," announces the development of an Ergonom-400 microscope, used by a German *Heilpraktiker*, or healer, Bernhard Muschlien, who paid a visit to Naessens's laboratory in 1985. While his microscope is apparently capable of achieving 25,000-fold magnification, its stated resolution is 100 nanometers (1000 angstroms), or several orders of magnitude less than the 150 angstroms developed with the somatoscope.*

In the July 1990 issue of *Popular Science*, an article, "Super Scopes," refers to an extraordinary new technology in microscopy engineered at Cornell University under the direction of Professor Michael Isaacson, and also in Israel. The technology uses not lenses but apertures smaller than the wave lengths of visible light to achieve high magnification. Isaacson is quoted as saying: "Right now, we can get about 40 nanometers (400 angstroms) of resolution," though he hopes to heighten that "power" to 100 angstroms "down the road." The 150 angstroms capacity built into Naessens's microscope over forty years ago still seems to lead the field.

Returning to the biography of Naessens, during the 1940s, the precocious young biologist began to develop novel anti-cancer products that had exciting new positive effects. The first was a confection he named "GN-24" for the initial letters of his first and last names, and for 1924, the year of his birth. Because official medicine had long considered cancerous cells to be basically "fermentative," in nature, reproducing by a process that, while crucial to making good wine from grape juice, produces no such salutary effect in the human body, Naessens's new product incorporated an "antifermentative" property. The train of his thinking, biologically or biochemically speaking, will not be here elaborated lest this account become too much of a "scientific treatise." What can be mentioned is that the new product, GN-24, sold in Swiss pharmacies, had excellent results when administered by doctors to patients with various forms of cancer.

As but one example of these results, Naessens cited to me the case of his own brother-in-law, on the executive staff

---

*One nanometer is one-billionth of a meter; one angstrom is ten-billionths of a meter, or one-tenth of a nanometer.

of the famed Paris subway system, the Métropolitain. In 1949, this relative, the husband of a now ex-wife's sister, was suffering through the terminal phase of stomach cancer and had been forced into early retirement. After complete recuperation from his affliction, he returned to work. Only recently, Naessens, who had lost contact with him for years, was informed that he was alive and well.

Another 1949 case was that of Germaine Laruelle, who was stricken with breast cancer plus metastases to her liver. A ghastly lesion that had gouged out the whole of the left section of her chest had caused her to go into coma when her family beseeched Naessens to begin his treatment. After recovering her health, fifteen years later, she voluntarily came to testify on behalf of Naessens, who, as we shall presently see, had been put under investigation by the French Ordre des Médecins (Medical Association). She also allowed press photographers to take pictures of the scars on the left side of her breast-denuded chest. In 1969, twenty years after her initial treatment, she died of a heart attack.

Seeking a more imposing weapon against cancer, Naessens next turned in the direction of a serum. This he achieved by hyperimmunizing a large draft horse as a result of injecting the animal with cancer-cell cultures, thus forcing it to produce antibodies in almost industrial quantities. Blood withdrawn from the horse's veins containing these antibodies, when purified, was capable of fighting the ravages of cancer. It proved to have therapeutic action far more extensive than that obtained by GN-24, and led to a restraint or reversal of the cancerous process, not only in cases of tumors but also with various forms of leukemia. Many patients clandestinely treated by their doctors with the new serum, called Anablast (*Ana*, "without," and *blast*, "cancerous cells"), were returned to good health.

One patient, successfully so treated, was to play a key role in Naessens's life. This was Suzanne Montjoint, then just past forty years of age, who, in 1960, developed a lump the size of a pigeon's egg in her left breast, which, over the next year, grew to become as large as a grapefruit. After the breast itself was surgically removed, Montjoint underwent a fifty-four-day course of radiation that caused horrible third-degree burns all over her chest. Within six months, she began to experience severe pain in her lower back.

Chemical examination revealed that the original cancer had spread to her fifth lumbar vertebra. More radiation not only could not alleviate the now excruciating pain, but caused a blockage in the functioning of her kidneys and bladder. When doctors told her husband she had only a week or so to live, Suzanne said to him, "I still have strength left to kill myself . . . but, tomorrow, I may not have it anymore."

Summoned by the husband, one of whose friends had told him about the biologist, Naessens began treating Madame Montjoint, who, by then, had lapsed into a semicoma. Within four days, all her pains disappeared and she had regained clarity of mind. By April 1962, after an examination of her blood at his microscope, Naessens declared that the somatid cycle in Suzanne Montjoint's blood had returned to normal. As she later told press reporters, "My recovery was no less than a resurrection!"

When these successful treatments, plus many others, came to the attention of French medical authorities, Naessens was twice brought before the bar of justice, first for the "illegal practice of medicine," next for the "illegal practice of pharmacy." On both occasions, he was heavily fined, his laboratory sealed, and most of its equipment confiscated, though, happily, he was able to preserve his precious microscope.

With all the harassment he was undergoing, while at the same time saving the lives of patients whose doctors could afford them little, or no, hope for recovery, Gaston Naessens was almost ready to emigrate from his mother country and find a more congenial atmosphere in which to pursue his work, with the privacy and anonymity that he had always cherished and still longs for. An opportunity to do so came when he was invited by doctors in a community that, if it was not a foreign country, might, like Québec in North America, seem to be one. The locale in question was the Mediterranean island of Corsica, whose inhabitants speak a dialect more akin to Italian than to French. With a long history of occupation by various invaders before it actually became part of the French Republic, its population has ever since been possessed of a revolutionary streak that, on occasion, fuels an urge toward secession from the "motherland."

In Corsica, Naessens established a small research laboratory in the village of Prunette, on the southwest tip of the island. What happened next, in all its full fury, cannot be told here. Reported in two consecutive issues of the leading Parisian illustrated weekly *Paris-Match*, the story would require, for any adequate telling, two or more chapters in a much longer book.

Suffice it to say that, having developed a cure for various forms of degenerative disease, Naessens saw his ivory tower invaded by desperate patients from all over the world who had learned of his treatment when a Scots Freemason, after hearing about it during a Corsican meeting with international members of his order, leaked them to the press in Edinburgh. Within a week, hundreds of potential patients were flying into Ajaccio, the island's capital, some of them from as far away as Czechoslovakia and Argentina.

The deluge immediately unleashed upon Naessens the wrath of the French medical authorities, who began a long investigation in the form of what is known in France as an *Instruction* — called in Québec an *Enquête préliminaire* — a kind of "investigative trial" before a more formal one.

All the "ins and outs" of this long jurisprudential process, thousands of pages of transcripts about which still repose in official Parisian archives, must, however regretfully, be left out of this narrative. Its denouement was that Gaston Naessens, together with key components of his microscope preserved on his person, left his native land in 1964 to fly to Canada, a country whose medical authorities he believed to be far more open to new medical approaches and horizons than those in France. His abrupt departure from the land of his birth was facilitated by a high-ranking member of France's top police organ, the *Sureté Nationale,* whose wife, Suzanne Montjoint, Naessens had successfully treated.

Hardly had Naessens set foot on Canadian soil than he was faced with difficulties, in fact a "scandal," almost as, if not just as, serious as the one he had just left behind.

During the French *Instruction* proceedings in 1964, one René Guynemer, a Canadian "war hero" of uncertain origin and profession, had accosted Naessens in his Paris domicile to beg him to come to Canada in order to treat his little three-year-old son, René Junior, who was dying of leukemia.

Though puzzled about a certain lack of "straightforwardness" in the supplicant, Naessens, ever willing to help anyone in distress, and with the approbation and assistance of the Canadian ambassador to France, immediately flew to Montréal, where he hoped, as agreed by Guynemer *père,* to be able to treat *fils* in complete discretion. Upon his arrival at Montréal's Dorval Airport, however, Naessens was aghast to see a horde of representatives of both the printed and visual media, creating, in anticipation of his arrival, what amounted to a virtual mob scene.

The Québec "Medical College" had, at the time, agreed, for "humanitarian" reasons, to allow the treatment of the Guynemer child, in spite of the fact that Anablast had not been licensed for use in Canada. Various tests, lasting for several weeks, were made on the product at Montréal's well-known microbiological Institut Armand Frappier to confirm the presence of gamma globulin in it, the presence of which purportedly thorough French examinations had failed to detect.

Virtually at death's door, the Guynemer child was said to have been given nine injections of Anablast. Naessens himself was never given official confirmation that the injections had actually been administered. Nor was he permitted to make any examination of the little patient's blood at his microscope, or even to meet him face to face. After the little boy succumbed, the Québec press exploded with stories that, in their luridness, matched the ones that had been appearing all over France after the Corsican "debacle."

Some of the mysteries of the "Guynemer connection" will likely never come to light. Only later did it become clear that the true name of the leukemic child's father was actually Lamer, a man who had claimed that, in past years, he had been an officer in the Royal Canadian Air Force and a "secret agent" attached to the French "underground" during World War II. To the Naessenses, the question has always remained: If he *was* an "agent," then for whom, or for what?

In the spring of 1965, Naessens journeyed to France for his trial. When he returned to Québec in the autumn of that year, he retired from the public scene to live incognito in Oka, a Montréal suburb, with a newfound friend, Hubert Lamontagne, owner of a business selling up-to-date electronic devices, whom he had met while looking for electrical components for his microscope in 1964. As a person skilled in electronics, Naessens was able to be of great assistance to his host, who also operated a large "repair shop" throughout the winter and the following summer, when, on tour with a troop of comedians, he was put in charge of solving all the acoustical problems in the many provincial cabarets and theaters hosting the troop's performances. Deprived, for several years, of any support to pursue his life goals, Naessens was constrained to utilize his skills as a "Mr. Fixit," able to repair almost anything from automobile engines to rectifiers.

In 1971, Naessens had a stroke of luck, perhaps the most important of his career, when, through another friend, he was introduced to, and came under the protective wing of, an "angel" who saw in Naessens the kind of genius he had for a long time been waiting to back.

That "angel" was the late David Stewart, head of Montréal's prestigious MacDonald-Stewart Foundation, which for many years had funded, as it still continues to fund, orthodox cancer research. Despondent about the recent death from cancer of a close friend, and in serious doubt that any of the cancer research he had so long supported would ever produce any solution, Stewart's guiding precept and motto was "In the search for a remedy for cancer, we shall leave no stone unturned." The philanthropist therefore decided *personally* to back Naessens's research. But after setting up a laboratory for the biologist on the Ontario Street premises of the well-known MacDonald Tobacco Company, which Stewart's father had inherited from its founder, tobacco magnate Sir William MacDonald, David Stewart came under such violent criticism by leaders of orthodox cancerology that he advised Naessens to move his research to a low-profile provincial retreat.

Having, by that time, established a "liaison" with his bride-to-be, Françoise Bonin, whose parents lived in Sherbrooke, Naessens was, by 1972, able to take over the elder Bonin's summer house on the banks of the Magog River in Rock Forest, "winterize" it, and establish a well-equipped laboratory in its basement. And there, the Naessenses, who were married in 1976, have ever since been located. Of his wife, Naessens has said to me, "She was persuaded from the very start about the intrinsic value of my research and at once saw the truth of it. Just as then, so now, years later, she continues her loyal assistance to get this truth out. Some ask if it's moral support. Yes, it could be called that. We have the same kind of attitudes about things. Both of us, for instance, believe that if something new produces good results, it's got to be pursued to the bitter end. This is not ambition, but moral honesty. When one gets to know her,

one realizes that she doesn't just repeat the things I think
and say, but is convinced about them because of what she
has seen and experienced."

Because legal restrictions applying to foundations and
their grants prevented David Stewart from transmitting monies directly to Naessens, the foundation director arranged for
them to be funneled via the Hôtel Dieu—a leading hospital
affiliated with the Université de Montréal that specializes
in orthodox cancer treatment and research. Accused by Augustin Roy as a "quack," Naessens has consequently had his
work modestly funded by checks made out by a hospital at
the heart of one of Canada's cancer establishment's most prestigious fund-granting institutions. No more anomalous a situation exists anywhere in the worldwide multibillion-dollar
cancer industry.

Given the importance of the foundation's assistance, it
is all the more curious that Augustin Roy had not made the
slightest mention of the foundation's loyal support of the biologist over the years. Instead, at a press conference held after Naessens's arrest to present traditional medicine's case
against Naessens, Roy, perhaps unknowingly, demonstrated
the "Catch-22" that any "alternative" medical, research, or
"frontier" scientist faces. Roy stated that if Naessens were
a "true" scientist he would have long since submitted his
results to proper authorities for check, but when asked by
journalists whether the Québec medical community had
thoroughly investigated the biologist's claims, Roy inscrutably
replied, "That's not our job." In answer to another reporter's
query about the assertions of many cancer patients that the
Naessens treatment had completely cured their affliction,
Roy added, "I just can't understand the *naivety and imbecil-
ity* of some people."

To get a more complete idea of the full impact of Roy's
attitude with respect to a brand new treatment and patients

benefiting from it, we here excerpt some of his additional statements made during an interview on McGill University's Radio Station in the summer of 1989.

When, to open the interview, Roy was asked his opinion about what the interviewer termed a "remarkable new anticancer product, 714-X," the medical administrator replied, "I have been aware of Monsieur Naessens for twenty-five years. In 1964, he arrived from France with a so-called cancer treatment, Anablast, the very same medicinal he's now using under another name—714-X."

That anyone in a position as elevated as Roy's could publicly propagate so obvious an error is surprising. For Anablast, which, as we have seen, is a serum, has nothing to do with 714-X, a biochemical product. Yet here was the head of the Québec medical establishment falsely stating that 714-X, developed over thirteen years in Canada, was nothing but the older French product bearing a new name, a statement tirelessly, and erroneously, repeated by journalists in the press.

As for Naessens himself, Roy told his radio audience: "That man's professional knowledge is equal to *zero!* You should know that he has, behind him, in France, an imposing, even 'heavy,' past involving serious judicial procedures and condemnations." It seems truly amazing that a doctor who, over a quarter of a century, had never met Naessens, or once visited his laboratory, or taken the trouble to investigate why hundreds of cancer patients had survived because of his new treatment, could so peremptorily reduce the biologist's knowledge to nil.

Was Roy really being impartial when he said, "I've got to be a bit careful because Naessens is currently under legal prosecution. . . . But the fact remains that he was in serious trouble with the French legal authorities. Let's just say he's a 'slick talker,' one who knows how to address an audience. But, I ask you, why is it that he's been working *in secret* for so long?" In asking this question, Roy was obviously not in the least ashamed to be adding a second error to the one he had already propagated. For the truth was, and is, that Naessens, far from having worked "in secret," has at all times—as I have repeatedly witnessed over the years—kept his laboratory open to "all comers" and has stood ready to discuss his research with any of them. "It's so obvious," Roy disparagingly continued, "that all this man's affirmations and allegations just don't have a leg to stand on. . . ."

"But," ingenuously interrupted his young interviewer, "haven't there been several people who have testified in writing, or on TV, that they've been cured by 714-X?"

Roy's unhesitating answer was breathtakingly categoric: *"No one's personal testimony has any value whatsoever!* All such testimonies are purely suggestive and anecdotal. Let's show a little common sense, after all! Common sense indicates that if Naessens had a real treatment for a malady such as cancer, it would have been *criminal* not to put it at the disposition of the whole world! I don't understand what he's up to, and I have even less understanding of those who go about publicizing his reputed treatment, which is pure *quackery.*" Given the hyperbole on Roy's part, one could well wonder what hope there might be for any kind of new discovery in the health field ever to become authorized, or even known. For years, Naessens had been assiduously, but unsuccessfully, trying to "put his discovery at the world's disposition."

Unabashed by the weight of her interviewee's authority, the interviewer was not loath to press in on Roy again: "There have, however, been certain doctors who have been most surprised at how terminal patients have been brought back to good physical shape with 714-X. Would that not make anyone eager to verify the facts with respect to those recovered patients?"

"Not at all!" Roy's rejoinder was a virtual explosion. "It's not my job, or that of the Medical Corporation, to check on *pseudocures* of that kind! So what, if two, three, four, or half

a dozen doctors, in their isolation, have something good to say in support of it? No matter where they come from, their statements are worthless!"

To get a countervailing idea of what Naessens might have said in rebuttal in Roy's presence, we shall next excerpt part of an interview with the biologist by the same interviewer on the same radio station a few days later.

"Gaston Naessens," she began, "is your 714-X really effective?"

Naessens: Absolutely! It builds up the immune system so that all the body's natural defenses can regain the upper hand. I don't make the claim in a void, because there are a lot of people around who were gravely ill with cancer who can now state they have gotten well due to my treatment.

Interviewer: If your product really works, why hasn't Dr. Roy been interested in doing an in-depth study of it? Does he know you at all?

Naessens: Many people have asked me both those questions. If you ask *him* the latter question, he will pull out a thick file on me and he'll tap it, and say, "Sure, I've known him since 1964." But the fact is he has *never* met me in person, *never* visited my lab, and *never* investigated my work! So, he is absolutely incapable of making any judgment whatsoever on whether that work has a solid foundation, or not!

In his lengthy reply, uninterrupted by the fascinated interviewer, Naessens, after a brief pause, began to reveal the essence of the difficult situation in which he had been placed over the years:

Naessens: Let's get to the heart of this matter! The medical community, on the one hand, and I, on the other, speak *completely different languages.* That anomaly connects to the important fact that *all approved anticancer therapies* are focused only on *cancer tumors and cancerous cells.* The reign-ing philosophy, medically speaking, is that a *cytolitic* (cell-killing) method must be used to destroy all cancer cells in a body stricken with that disease.

But I, on the contrary, have developed a therapy based on what has been called the body's whole *terrain*! To under-stand that, you have to realize that, every day, our bodies produce cancerous cells in no great amount. It's our healthy *immune system* that gets rid of them. My 714-X allows a weakened, or hampered, immune system to come back to full strength, so that it can do its proper job!

If medical "experts" pronounce my product worthless, it might even be admitted that, in terms of their own scien-tific philosophy, they are making some sense. This is largely because, when they examine my product for any *cytotoxic* effect it might have, they find none!

Interviewer: Is the Medical Corporation interested in sit-ting down and talking with you, or running tests to verify your product?

Naessens: No! Because they firmly believe that any suc-cess it might have is due to some kind of "psychological" effect, and they say that the product itself contains nothing that could possibly be of benefit.

Interviewer: Where did they get that idea?

Naessens: It seems that, with officialdom, it's always a case of misinformation, or of bad faith. If this whole affair were limited to patients I've successfully treated, patients who might have remained silent, I would still have small hope that my research will one day be recognized. But, now, a cru-cial turning point has been reached. I'm back in the interna-tional limelight. My arrest, incarceration, and indictment are important if only because, immediately following them, peo-ple "in the know" have begun to take action on my behalf. That being so, the medical community's negative reaction is no longer the only, or the dominant, one! It may be too bad that all this has to be thrashed out not in a scientific forum, but in a court of law. But that's the way it is. In my upcoming trial, many of my patients' cases will be examined, one by one, and exposed in full detail, in the courtroom! So the medical "authorities" will no longer be the sole judges.

After continuing on with this theme for several minutes longer, Naessens came to a firm conclusion: "I wouldn't want you to think that I'm even trying to boast when I say that my work represents a *brand new horizon in biology!* I have found a successful way of adjusting a delicate biological mechanism. I have no pretensions beyond that! If I can be of service to anyone, my laboratory is always open."

Chapter 3
The Birth of Public Support

*Whatever the judgment of the courts in the case of
biologist Gaston Naessens, the affair cannot but raise
fundamental issues about health care that ultimately
society itself must resolve. Is it reasonable that the
medical establishment continues to exercise a monopoly
in the field of health care?*

Ed Bantey, columnist,
The Montréal Gazette, 2 July 1989

Some of the deeper, and broader, issues behind the trial, as
brought out by the two McGill University radio interviews,
were concisely summed up, and bolstered, on 2 July 1989,
when *The Gazette,* Montréal's leading English-language newspaper, ran one of the many *Beau Dimanche* (Beautiful Sun-
day) columns written by Ed Bantey, a veteran commentator
on important social issues. Far from pulling any punches, the
article's title, both a challenge and an accusation, was as direct
as a prize fighter's roundhouse right to the jaw: "It's Time to
Look at the Medical Establishment's Monopoly."

Bantey asked many pertinent and probing questions,
among them: "Should we give orthodox medicine *carte
blanche* to block recourse to alternative therapies that offer
even limited promise?" "Given its inflexibly adamant stand
against women's pleas to allow midwives, rather than male
obstetricians, to birth their babies," the *Gazette* columnist
continued, "it is obvious that vested interests, who view their
privileges as threatened, are mainly concerned to resist any
change in the *status quo.*"

All of Bantey's declarative and interrogative statements were brought into sharp focus when, on 27 June, the demonstrators, some of the "naive imbeciles" to whom Roy had referred and their friends and relatives, trooped downhill from the courthouse to the Wellington Hotel, where a newly formed "Committee for the Defense of Gaston Naessens" hosted its first press conference.

The event opened with committee president Ralph (Raoul) Ireland outlining what would be presented. A native Québecer, fluent in French and English, Ireland, no braggart, did not make known his own interesting background. Great grandson of James Redmond, founder of the Irish Republican Army (IRA); son of a distinguished Canadian engineer; one of the "unofficial," but actual, founders of the world-known Greenpeace movement that fights for causes as disparate as the rights of rivers to be free of pollution and the right of dolphins and whales to be free of massacre by humans; speaker of the *Cant* (Irish Gypsy) language—Ralph Ireland, in early 1989, raised money and opened Canada's only quartz crystal mine in Bonsecours, a spot on the road a little over thirty kilometers northwest of Sherbrooke.

Explaining to the press that some dozen former cancer patients, treated by Naessens after their doctors had given them little or no hope of recovery, would tell their stories, Ireland added, "Everything they say can be meticulously documented by their medical records."

For two hours, the patients, young and old, offered their stories to the assembled representatives of the press, radio, and television. Among the most poignant was that of sixty-four-year-old Roland Caty, who, while in charge of the construction of a new university in the tiny African country of Rwanda, was diagnosed as having an adenosarcoma—a particularly lethal tumor that develops rapidly—in his prostate. After his doctors advised him to have all of his sexual organs ablated, Caty, knowing that so horrible an operation would be unlikely to preserve what was left of his body, refused the dictum. His surgeon, bluntly and coldly, told him he was "crazy" and that, without such an operation, he would be dead within three months.

"Well, I knew damn well that, if I submitted to that butchery," Caty told the press conference, "I wouldn't last much longer than three months! I was fortunate to know Gaston Naessens, learn of his 714-X treatment, and become one of the first, if not *the* first, to take it. Because I had to go back to my job in Africa, I also learned how to make the injections myself, into the lymph node in my groin. And here I am testifying to you eleven years after I got well!"

Caty's testimony was followed by that of Belgian-born Jean-Hubert Eggerman, who had had an operation for intestinal cancer only to find the affliction had metastasized into his liver. "I began the Naessens treatments on February 14th of this year [1989]," he declared, "and now I feel fine. Before that, I was exposed to chemotherapy, even though the doctors who prescribed it gave me no hope of cure whatsoever. The 'chemo' made me sick as a dog! I could go into all the gory details of it, but I won't. I told my wife, 'I just can't stand it anymore! Let things take their course!' I decided to quit . . . to give up . . . to die! Then I was introduced to Naessens."

Eggerman and other witnesses described how they had been harassed by undercover investigative agents employed by the Medical Corporation, who had invaded their privacy either by incessantly telephoning to try to pry information out of them, or actually invading their homes, without search warrants, to rifle through desk drawers and closets in search of Naessens's vials of 714-X and other evidence. "How come this kind of harassment is permitted and condoned?" Eggerman was almost shouting. "How the hell did these 'goons' get my name or my confidential medical file? We're not living in Stalinist Russia or Nazi Germany here! We're in Canada! When the hell is all this going to stop? When am I and the

rest of us going to win the right to be treated as we see fit?"
All of which, like Ed Bantey's article, pretty much got to the
very heart of the true nature of what the "Naessens Affair,"
as it had come to be called, was all about.

Another particularly moving affidavit was that of Raoul
Poissant, whose tongue and larynx had been surgically excised. Left to die by his doctors, he was introduced by friends
to Naessens and recovered after 714-X treatment. Poissant
was forced to write his testimony onto a legal pad while
another younger recovered cancer patient read it aloud word
for word as the ink was pouring from his pen.

Next on the microphone was Bernard Baril, a thirty-
three-year-old Québec-born restaurant and catering consultant, who, when working in Paris, had been tested positive
for HIV (Human Immunodeficiency Virus), the prime vec-
tor in AIDS. Almost breaking down, Baril described how, after cancerous growths began to fill his mouth and attack his
palate, doctors at the Montréal General Hospital had told him
he was so far gone as to not be worth treating.

Almost unable to take nourishment, Baril lay in his bed,
his weight declining from 155 to 115 pounds, until, in April
1988, a friend introduced him to Naessens. Within three
months, Baril began witnessing the miraculous disappearance
of his lesions. Choking back a sob, he told the press conference, "Look at me! I now weigh 170 pounds! I feel entirely
fit! Don't I look in the pink of health?"

It was only in the summer of 1990 that the full facts
taken from the dossier of Bernard Baril were finally made
available. They reveal that this AIDS-afflicted patient had,
on 3 March 1988, been diagnosed as having a cancerous
growth, Karposi's sarcoma, on his palate, together with cancerous invasions of his lymphatic system. A biopsy consisting of a piece of tissue measuring $1 \times 1 \times 0.2$ cm. was submitted in toto, meaning that the whole of a cancerous growth
was cut out. Another piece of tissue measuring $0.5 \times 0.2 \times 0.3$

cm. was also submitted in toto. The tumor received a IV-D, or "extremely advanced," classification.

Baril refused all conventional treatment. When he finally began 714-X treatment, his weight had dropped from a normal 165 pounds to 115 pounds! This treatment began on 3 June 1988. Three days later, the tumor on the palate had reappeared and, by 22 June, measured 0.8 × 0.2 × 0.3 cm. Baril was a little discouraged.

But, by 11 July, he began to become encouraged when the tumor, beginning to decrease in size, measured 0.6 × 0.2 × 0.3 cm. During the next six months, it *completely disappeared*. On 29 March 1990, a reevaluation by Dr. Tyler, the same physician who had first seen Baril, indicated that "there was no tumor present but only a discolored zone measuring 1.0 × 0.5 cm. A blood test revealed that Baril's blood parameters were normal." In the summer of 1990, Baril was, to quote him, "at the top of his form," and had no symptoms of cancer whatsoever.

After the press conference disbanded at the Wellington, a crowd, now swelled to more than two hundred people, gathered in the same hotel's "Flamingo Room," a nightclub with a raised dancing floor that had suddenly become the site of a daytime reception and rally.

Defense Committee President Ireland rose again to consolidate the fighting spirit of the demonstrators. "We count on every one of you to help in presenting the truth about an avatar of medicine, *true medicine*," his voice boomed out in Québec-accented French. "It's doers, not thinkers, who really accomplish something in life, and get things to change. Naessens is one of those doers! So what about the rest of us? As for me, I am not afraid to speak out against the injustice of medical monopoly. We're supposed to be living in a *free country* and it's to be hoped that our beloved Canada will remain free from every point of view, that no gates into freedom's city, medical or otherwise, will ever be locked in our nation!"

Because the 27 June court hearing had merely postponed any judicial opinion as to the furtherance of Naessens's trial date until 14 July, when that date arrived a second demonstration and press conference were held in Sherbrooke.

This time, as reported by veteran court reporter Jacques Lemoine, in a Sherbrooke *Tribune* front-page story, it appeared that Naessens was garnering impressive judicial, medical, and international support in his battle against the Québec Medical Corporation.

In front of a throng of more than two hundred people, Naessens's attorney, Conrad Chapdelaine, a diminutive man of no more than five feet six inches in height, but with a visage that calmly suggested a personage of great inner stature, took the microphone to announce that, during the brief court session, the presiding judge had ruled that previous strictures imposed on Naessens would be lifted, to allow him to regain the same freedom of action he had enjoyed before charges had been brought against him. "This represents a real victory," Chapdelaine cheered his audience of Naessens's supporters, but he also cautioned that the really important, and crucial, battle would be trial before a jury to take place some time in late October or early November.

Seated under klieg lights at the press conference was a panel of notables who, one by one, asserted that Naessens, far from being a know-nothing or a quack, was a first-rank, if hardly known, pioneer of brand new medical research.

Among them was Florianne Piers, M.D., a Belgian, who said she had taken the time to come over to the rally because she had, over a four-month period, begun to treat seven cancer patients with Naessens's 714-X. "The product prolonged the lives, and eased the deaths, of two terminally afflicted patients," announced Piers, "and has allowed the other five, who came to me with seriously advanced cancerous states, to see every one of their symptoms disappear and to take up their lives as if they had never incurred the disease." Asked whether

Belgian medical authorities might not impose sanctions against her for using an "unapproved" medicinal, such as revoking her hospital privileges, Piers boldly answered that, if that turned out to be the case, she would treat her patients at home.

Next to take the microphone on Naessens's behalf was a soft-spoken general practitioner, Raymond Keith Brown, M.D., from New York City, where, for some time, he had worked on problems of cancer research at the world-famous Sloan-Kettering Institute. Brown was author of a book entitled *AIDS, Cancer and the Medical Establishment* (New York: Robert Speller, 1986), the first publication to print micrographs of what Naessens had discovered.

In a soft Virginian drawl, Brown declared that he was truly convinced that Naessens, whose work he had been following since 1975, was a genius. He specifically referred to the case of one of his own patients, whom he had most successfully treated with 714-X for a cancer of the pancreas that had proved unamenable to any other form of treatment. Though it should not be thought of as a "panacea," Brown added, 714-X certainly deserved to take its place in the armory of weapons available to official medicine.

As trenchant as were Brown's supportive words, it was left to Walter Clifford, who, before founding his own research firm in Colorado Springs, Colorado, had worked for many years as a bacteriological expert for the U.S. Army, to tell the central, hidden, and utter truth about what was really transpiring behind the scenes in Naessens's struggle with the "Medical College." Commenting on the general unwillingness of the mainstream medical industry to support alternative research, Clifford courageously averred: "Sad as it is, my scientific colleagues and I have found to our bitter dismay that, if you don't 'toe the company line,' medical pundits don't even want to know about your discoveries, whatever they might be!"

As the patients' press conference was going on, Naessens was also gaining support of a different kind. Among many letters in Naessens's defense that were pouring in to the *Route de l'Église* office of Gil Rémillard, Québec's minister of justice, was one signed by Renaud Vignal, who, before his 1987 appointment as French ambassador to the Seychelles, had served for three years as his country's consul general in Québec. Vignal wrote that he had been profoundly shocked to learn that "a man whom my wife, Anne, and I hold in highest esteem," had been detained and was under criminal investigation.

Vignal explained to Rémillard that, in 1984, his wife had undergone an examination to determine why she had not been able to have a baby. To her horror, the exam revealed that she was afflicted with a form of leukemia so lethal that doctors in three countries (Canada, France, and the United States) had given her not more than three to five years to live. Other than "maintenance" chemotherapy, they could recommend no treatment to save her life except bone-marrow grafts for which there was no compatible donor.

Vignal wrote that, in their despair, he and his wife had the luck to meet Naessens. Anne underwent treatment with 714-X by intralymphatic injection. As to the result, the ambassador stated in his letter:

> My wife is alive five years after her initial diagnosis and, in spite of the fact that a host of physicians told her she never could have a child—due to protracted and uninterrupted chemotherapy—we have just had a magnificent little healthy son in a birth that, lying outside any "medical" explanation not to be considered a "miracle," we can only attribute to the gentle administrations of our dear friend, Gaston Naessens.

The Vignalses' son is named Gaspard, the first three letters of his name intentionally chosen to match the first three letters of Gaston's.

Supporting Vignal's letter was another from Gaston Mialaret, professor of education at the Université de Caen, in Normandy, who had also taught at the Université du Québec in Trois-Rivières, served as director for international education at UNESCO in Geneva, Switzerland, and been awarded honorary doctorates by the universities of Sherbrooke (Québec), Ghent (Belgium), and Lisbon (Portugal).

"I have known Gaston Naessens for over twenty years," wrote Mialaret to Rémillard.

There comes a time when friendship must be publicly expressed, especially when it's a case of a man's honor. I know that his research findings are upsetting certain ideas normally accepted in the world of medicine and science. Whether he is right or not, scientifically speaking, he is an unquestionably honest man whose only aim is to help and cure the ills of humanity.

My conscience cannot accept, without revulsion, that he be treated as a swindler and a charlatan: an affirmation that dishonors those who make it and reveals their hatred or lack of objectivity. I have confidence in your country's justice and am therefore convinced that not alone the letter, but the spirit, of its laws will take into account the many positive aspects of Naessens's work.

Finally, Gaston Naessens himself addressed the assembly. His gray jacket bedecked with a spray of white carnations, he spoke with quiet confidence and humility, which all who have interacted with him have come, like Ambassador Vignal, to recognize as two of his chief character traits. "As I go over in my mind the events of the last forty years," he told his loyal supporters, "I believe I can, without boastfulness, and looking you all straight in the eye, say: mission accomplished." Even with the difficult legal battles still to come, Naessens expressed no regrets: "For if there were in this room, or anywhere, a single patient whose life was extended for one, two, five, or ten years due to my treatment," he concluded, "I would be prepared to go on the long and difficult trek I have made all over again."

Part Two
Battle in Court

Chapter 4
The Trial Begins

[F]or no great discovery has ever been immediately accepted. Rather, in medicine it seems that the reverse is true, and everyone must go through a period of trial and even censure before what seems the obvious truth is recognized generally. . . . But such slow acceptance prevents the real discoveries from being known and widely accepted earlier, and many lives are thus sacrificed needlessly.

Frank Slaughter, *Immortal Magyar: Semmelweiss, Conqueror of Childbed Fever*

"Silence! Debout, s'il vous plaît!" With that cry from the bailiff, all in the tiny courtroom stood as Judge Jean-Louis Péloquin, in his black robe and white dicky draped with a crimson red stole, walked in to take his seat on the bench.

The trial of Gaston Naessens had begun. No, it was definitely not "Perry Mason," in either the setting or the atmosphere. First of all, the court was arranged not to heighten, but to lessen, any drama. Witnesses took the "stand"—there was no witness box, so they literally *stood* at floor level—facing front, with their backs to the spectators. Since no loudspeakers were in use, spectators were hard put to hear their testimony or even the questions of the two opposing lawyers.

Jacques Lemoine, reporter for Sherbrooke's *Tribune*, kindly made room for me at the press table, directly behind the prosecutor's table, thus allowing me easily to hear nearly everything that was said, and affording me a view of Gaston Naessens and his defense lawyer, Conrad Chapdelaine.

Chapdelaine, in whom Gaston and Françoise Naessens seem to place great confidence, is a short wiry man with a head of thick jet-black hair and a walrus mustache to match.

Were he not wearing the black robe and paper-white shirt-front and stiff collar, *de rigueur* for Québécois attorneys while in court, he might seem to be not so much a member of the legal profession as a tough cavalry colonel in the horde of a Tamerlane or a Genghis Khan. The dark skin of his face is set with eyes that frequently flash with a foxy look as if he were about to uncork a "surprise." All in all, he seems to radiate quiet confidence with no hint of arrogance or boastfulness.

One could gain the opposite impression of the mien of the Crown's prosecutor, Claude Melançon, whose "styled" brush-cut hairdo and an often supercilious expression reflected a kind of effetely disdainful attitude. Melançon is taller by two or three inches than Chapdelaine, but that seemed to provide him no advantage.

Then there was the jury of eleven, five men and six women, mostly "simple" people—hardly an intellectual or sophisticate among them. Was this good? Probably. For they were likely to weigh matters with values and impressions untrammeled by too much "knowledge." The age bracket went from the twenties to the sixties, or beyond. A few had perplexed, one or two even oafish, expressions; I focused on a woman with protruding eyes and wondered if she realized that she might hold the life of a man in her hands.

As the proceedings got under way, I found myself having to "cock my ears" to grasp all that was being said. Though I had been in the small French-speaking enclave of North America off and on for more than three months, I still had not fully adapted to the French-Canadian accent, which is difficult to describe to anyone who does not know standard French. There are unfamiliar diphthongs that have a weird ring: *chaise* (chair), for instance, comes out as *"sha-ezz,"* as if it were two syllables, instead of *"shehzz"* as in France. A Frenchman educated to speak standard American English—the kind spoken by radio or TV news announcers—would have the same difficulty in the Deep South, where a word such as the proper noun Anne is voiced as *"Ah-yenne."*

From the very outset, it might seem that not one but two trials were taking place or, more specifically, that the Crown prosecutor and his adversary were fighting, the one on a narrow fencing ground with an épée, against a single, and less skilled, opponent, the other in a vast arena with a mace, against a small legion of veteran soldiers.

In his opening remarks, Crown prosecutor Melançon set the tone of his case by making things as simple as possible. The main, and most serious, allegation on which he single-mindedly focused was Naessens's supposedly false promise to cure completely a patient afflicted with breast cancer that had spread to her lymph system. By offering her treatment, unrecognized by medicine and unlicensed by health authorities, he had significantly contributed to her death and was, therefore, an accessory to what amounts to murder. Bluntly reducing the whole dire matter to a single sentence, Melançon intoned sternly: "What we shall prove is that Naessens *lied*, and *knew* he was lying."

The hopefully fatal one-time thrust of the épée!

Though judge, jury, and spectators would have to wait, interminably it seemed, for thirteen days of meandering, often highly technical, testimony by prosecution witnesses, a lot of it full of medical jargon and often seasoned with irrelevancies, to at last hear how the defense would counter it, we might as well, right at this point, offset the prosecutor's simplistic case by summarizing what Chapdelaine was to put forward in his own opening remarks. "We shall try, as modestly as possible," his tone was almost hushed, "to present to you the substance of our client's whole *oeuvre* and make clear that that substance lies outside and beyond medicine as traditionally practiced. In so doing, we will also detail for you what he has accomplished over the years, how he has developed his research and interacted with people, and what have been his contributions to medicine and science."

The hopefully decimating, whirling, mace!

A trial, the transcript of which runs to thousands of pages, is not easy to sum up in space as limited as that afforded in this book. Our task is to capture its essence, to cut film footage, taken over days, down to an incisive two-hour cinema drama.

Introducing the case for the prosecution was Luc Grégoire, a beefily handsome member of the Québec *Sureté*, who, throughout the trial, sat at the prosecutor's table to help him with his documentation. On 13 December 1984, Grégoire led a search of Naessens's house and laboratory, accompanied by two "investigative commissioners" of the Medical Corporation, two other representatives of which sat sporadically in court throughout the trial, listening with dour faces to what witnesses, particularly those for the defense, had to say and, presumably, reporting it back to Augustin Roy. The search party was mainly looking for a pair of medical dossiers, the most important one of which was that of Madame Langlais, the patient to whose death Naessens had supposedly contributed. What they sought in her file was supportive material to back up an eight-page "Declaration" elicited from, and signed on 12 November 1984 by, her husband, Marcel, at the corporation's instigation. It was to this document that the prosecutor repeatedly referred, so much so that I gained a strong impression that, had he not had access to it, his case would have been extremely "thin."

Three assertions stood out in the declaration on which Melançon heavily relied to bolster his proof. The first was Langlais's statement that "everyone addressed Naessens as 'Doctor,' and my wife and I took this title to mean 'Doctor of Medicine,' and, in particular, 'cancer-specialist.'" At no time in his life has Naessens ever allowed himself to be called a "doctor"—in fact, he has taken pains to deny it whenever the term was used.

The second assertion to which Langlais put his signature was in the declaration's wording: "He promised us that, after the first series of treatments, her cancer would be completely cured." While, as the defense would make abundantly clear, Naessens at no time made such a promise to anyone, this statement, as we have seen, was used by the prosecution as a cornerstone in the edifice of its argument.

The third glaring assertion in Langlais's submission to the Medical Corporation—whether willingly offered or extracted from him—was that, during the course of Madame Langlais's treatment, "Naessens kept assuring us that she was making real progress." The defense would ultimately convince the jury that this was an utter distortion of the truth.

The search party that raided Naessens's house and laboratory was after bigger game than just the Langlais dossier, as evidenced by their seizure of some 150 additional medical files in Naessens's possession. But because, to their sure dismay, they could find nothing incriminating in them, they were returned to Naessens a few months later.

Also seized were five vials containing the biologist's 714-X product, each of them clearly labeled: "For Export: 5 ml. dose vial, 714-X, *Camphorminium Chloride.* For Intralymphatic Injection Only. Experimental Product for Sole Use by the Medical Corps. Experimental Center for Biological Research in the Eastern Townships, Inc., Rue Fontaine, Rock Forest, Québec."

The wording on the label is important if only to show that its precise meaning was distorted when, on 2 June 1989, only a week following Naessens's arrest, *Santé et Bien-Être Canada* (Health and Welfare, Canada, or HWC) issued an official bulletin: "Warning Concerning 714-X, A Fraudulent Anti-Cancer Therapeutic Product." "The HWC's Office for the Protection of Health," the bulletin's text began, "has today alerted the population to the fact that a product called 714-X, an injectable preparation, is offered as an anti-cancer treatment. Anyone who has procured this preparation is advised not to use it and to throw it out forthwith." Going on to list what was printed on the label, HWC included only that part of it referring to: "714-X . . . Camphorminium Chloride . . . Intralymphatic Injection . . . Experimental Product . . . For Export," but omitted the key phrase "for Sole Use by the Medical Corps."

To this key "sin of omission," the bulletin, in its eagerness to condemn a new product in the eyes of the medical community and the public at large, next added a "sin of commission": "The self-administration by injection, which is the method indicated on the label, presents grave risks." How could Canadian officials, responsible for the health of all citizens, have intentionally informed them about a supposed method that nowhere appeared on the label itself? The answer to this question has, at this writing, not yet been clarified and, until it is, one may justifiably ask whether such officials did not grossly overstep their mandate in seeking to get rid of a product that might well be of enormous assistance to cancer patients.

And that was not the last distortion in the bulletin, which went on to read: "According to the laboratory analysis made by the Office for the Protection of Health, 714-X contains only camphor and not—as is written on the label—any *camphorminium chloride*. There is no scientific proof of these chemical products, nor of their effectiveness, in cancer treatment. The Office, in collaboration with the Québec *Sureté*, is carrying out an investigation on the fraudulent sale and distribution of the product in question. All persons who have used any 714-X should receive appropriate medical care."

Though Melançon would wait until the very last day of his presentation to introduce, as his last witness, the Office for the Protection of Health's chemist, Michel Lefebvre, who said he had determined the chemical composition of 714-X, we shall take up the problem right at this point. This is because 714-X had, through willful distortion of the kind illustrated above, been falsely branded as "an aqueous solution tinged only with a trace of camphor," or, worse still, "nothing but water," and therefore of no therapeutic value whatsoever.*

Though Naessens had repeatedly been accused of inventing the name "camphorminium chloride" out of whole cloth as it were, the facts are otherwise. This name was given to the product not by its inventor, but by one of Montréal's oldest and most respected patent firms, Robic et Robic (founded 1888), after one of that firm's associates, Thierry Ohrlac, both a chemist and a patent lawyer, had completed investigative work on it with the cooperation, among others, of the United States Patent Office in Washington, D.C.

The key molecule in the preparation, both novel and complex, was synthesized to include nitrogen compounds that are crucial to its functioning.** Together with the name

---

*The false allegation went far beyond the frontiers of Canada. While in France, in the mid-1980s, I was present during a virtual TV "blitz" on prime time that focused on the *Affaire Naessens*, with the media's accenting, with gleeful *schadenfreude*, news from Canada that Naessens was again in trouble with the law. I well remember how clips from the films he had made of the somatid cycle at the microscope were broadcast to the French nation while the commentator derisively announced that what viewers were watching were no more than "animated cartoons." When I called a French Nobel Laureate in Microbiology, whom I had met at a conference in Pugwash, New Brunswick, fifteen years before, to ask him what he thought might be the effective ingredients in Naessens's product, he angrily replied, "C'est de l'eau, Monsieur, rien que de l'eau, vous m'entendez bien? C'est tout ce que j'ai à vous dire!" (It's water, Monsieur, nothing but water, do you get me? That's all I have to say to you!) And, with that, he hung up.

**The nitrogen is carried to tumor cells so avid for the element they have been called "nitrogen traps." By flooding the body with nitrogen and thus sating the cancerous cells, the same action also suppresses a secretion that, as Naessens discovered, paralyzes the immune system.

assigned by the patent firm, the molecule's chemical composition, as illustrated in a formula, was officially accepted on 16 February 1980 by the Canadian Patent Office, and thenceforth authorized, if not for domestic use, at least for export. So, far from being a "quack" product clandestinely circulated by a "charlatan," it had won a *status* as defined by the above-cited governmental actions.

When the government chemist, Lefebvre, called as a prosecution witness, claimed that his analyses had revealed 714-X to be only an aqueous solution of camphor—"camphor and water"—his testimony was destroyed under cross-examination, during which he was forced to admit that, had he run other tests, he would indeed have found the important nitrogen-associated components.

Precisely at noon on the first day of the trial, Judge Péloquin, who had been looking at his watch to get the timing exact, announced a lunch break, as he would on every succeeding day of the trial.

When court resumed session in the afternoon, Grégoire, under cross-examination by Chapdelaine, was asked whether he had gone back a second time to search the Naessenses' premises in 1985 or 1986. His reply: "To my best recollection, I did not!" This answer seemed to establish for the jury that no thorough-going attempt had been made by the police organ either to inventory, or assess, all of the elaborate equipment in Naessens's laboratory which, in turn, implied a total lack of interest in his research methods and technique.

Chapter 5
The Surgeon
and the Somatid

A cancerology "big boss" told us quite recently, "Watch out! You're straying from the main track. If you get too far outside the system, the products you've developed, as good as they are or might be, will never have a chance."
                    Monique and Mirko Beljanski,
              French cancer researchers, *Health Confiscated*

An essential aspect of the prosecution's case, and one of the main themes of the trial, began to emerge with the appearance on the stand of a ranking Québec physician and cancer surgeon, Lorenzo Haché, M.D., who had done all his medical studies in English, interned in Toledo, Ohio, and spent four years working at the renowned Mayo Clinic in Minnesota, before returning to practice at home. Madame Langlais's family doctor had recommended her to Haché when she was diagnosed with breast cancer.

As its star witness, Haché was taken step by step by the prosecution into all the technical, often gruesome, details of a cancer case. There was the mammography, the clinical test and exams, the description of "dripping" from a breast lesion with a tumor in it measuring 4.5 centimeters in diameter, a swollen lymph ganglion under one armpit indicating that the cancer had metastasized, and on and on. In short, almost anyone might, without any sophisticated medical knowledge, infer that Madame Langlais, with an advanced stage of cancer, was doomed.

But how far advanced? That was the crucial question. If she had no hope of recovery, by any means, then Naessens could hardly, at least not fairly, be implicated in her death.

Rather, his treatment, unorthodox as it might be, could be seen as a "last chance," however remote. The prosecution, therefore, placed high hopes in Haché to state unequivocally that Langlais did, in fact, stand an excellent chance to recover by orthodox treatments. And Melançon got him to intimate, rather than to firmly aver, that, had she submitted to surgical ablation of her breast, then, maybe, she could have stood a chance of cure.

But, under cross-examination, Chapdelaine extracted from the surgeon the additional admission that the patient indeed did have a cancer-infected lymph node and that, consequently, there "might be other metastases in her body that could not be detected or analyzed."

There was no question that Langlais would ever have submitted to Haché's surgery, as even her husband's declaration to the Medical Corporation made abundantly clear. Her fear of such an operation, and of hospitals in general, was what had made her opt for Naessens's treatment. But the lengths to which surgeons will go to "cut," to force patients under their knives, was brought out when Haché said he was most surprised that Langlais had not appeared in his hospital on the assigned date to have her breast surgically removed, and particularly by his adding, "We often send out police to locate such reluctant patients."

Another symbol of the tie between medicine and law enforcement?

The dapperly dressed and groomed surgeon was inveigled to further expatiate on details of orthodox cancer treatment by surgery, radiation, and chemotherapy, the so-called cut, burn, or poison techniques. This treatment, Haché admitted, was often no more than "preventative" (used to stop, but not to cure, the inevitable progress of a cancerous condition) or "palliative" (used to decrease pain). The sum total of his remarks seemed to suggest that treatment might help, but the statistics he provided cast strong doubt. At one point, Haché came to the conclusion that, according to such "statistics" Langlais had a "thirty-five percent" chance of full recovery through standard treating procedures.

It seemed to me that even the jury, wholly untrained in medicine, could see through this "numbers game," protractedly played out by the prosecutor to bolster his proof that Langlais would, in fact, have had a real chance of being cured had she, instead of turning to Gaston Naessens, submitted to the surgeon's interventions. Against this backdrop, I could not help wondering what was really going on in the minds of each of the six women on the eleven-person jury as all the horrors of breast cancer were being spelled out.

Perhaps feeling that his witness was not making as compelling a case as he had hoped, Melançon, apparently oblivious to the fact that it ran completely against his best interest, next turned his line of questioning to a subject that was also central to the trial's overall theme and, in so doing, began dragging Haché into deeper water. He asked the doctor to explain to the jury exactly what the body's lymph system was, and how it functioned. After briefly describing the circulatory system, its arteries, veins, and their own functioning, the doctor went on to say that the lymph system, which performs a "drainage" role, is made up of tiny canal-like vessels interspaced and interconnected with ganglia, or nodes, many of which, if cancer afflicted, are surgically removed, whether or not they are "palpable," or swollen.

It was during the last hour of the court session—after the usual afternoon fifteen-minute coffee break—that it became plain *why* Melançon had brought up the lymph system in the first place. Dr. Haché was shown the label on one of the vials containing Naessens's 714-X product and asked to read aloud for the jury the words: "for intralymphatic injection." "Could such a product as 714-X actually be intralymphatically injected?" asked the prosecutor, bound and determined to prove that such was not the case, and certain the surgeon would uphold him.

But the doctor hesitated. Well, certain dyes were sometimes so injected, he replied, but it was a very "difficult process" accomplishable only by "experts," and then only when supported with local anesthesia, because it was otherwise extremely painful. Haché further maintained that the same process could not be accomplished without first making an incision through the skin and that, even then, it was often impossible to find a lymph canal, or node, into which the injection might be made.

Under insistent and specific questioning, Haché, as if seeking to be shed of the matter, firmly asserted, "Lymph injection is *never done* in any hospital because it's *impossible!*"

Right there, it seemed to me that Haché had stumbled badly. As Françoise Naessens put her reaction to me following the court session: "In light of Haché's statement, I think things are going very well indeed!" Meaning, of course, for her husband, Gaston. Implied, by her remark, was that the defense had, probably unwittingly, laid bare what Françoise termed the ignorance of a veteran physician and surgeon when it came to the matter of intralymphatic injection. If such an "expert" could make so gross an error, and the jury could be made to see it as an error by the defense attorney, then how could his testimony on the matter possibly stand up?

We have seen, in the first part of this book, how easy it was for Roland Caty, with no medical training whatsoever, not only to learn, within hours, how to inject 714-X into a lymph system, but to self-inject it into his own lymph system. But here was Haché asserting such injection was next to impossible.

And that was not the only time Haché stumbled. For, as Haché's testimony was drawing to a close, the prosecutor showed him Langlais's medical dossier and, drawing his attention to its fourth page, specifically asked him to look at

a line reading: " . . . examination of somatids in the blood."
Stepping backward half a pace and waving his hand for emphasis, Melançon asked, in mock triumph, "Have you ever
heard of so-called somatids, doctor?"

Again Haché hesitated. "Well . . . no," he finally replied,
then added, "But since I did my medical studies in the English language, I could be ignorant of the term. . . . I seem
to recall having seen it somewhere in a French book. . . . I
can't recall which. . . . "

When next asked about other forms in the sixteen-stage
cycle, also found in patient Langlais's blood examination, the
surgeon said he had never heard the terms *asci* or *levurids*
(yeastlike forms) and stated categorically that, whatever they
were, they would *never* be seen in the blood or its red cells.
About several other forms in the cycle, Haché stated exasper-
atedly: "I don't know what they can possibly refer to!" And,
a moment later: "We don't even know what kind of examination Naessens is making here!"

And that's the point—the crux of the whole matter. A
question sprang into my mind as soon as those words were out
of the surgeon's mouth: If they *don't know* . . . the doctors . . .
then why don't they *find out*? Before passing something off as
worthless, something they have never taken a minute, let alone
an hour, to investigate, why don't they take the trouble to look
into it? Are they not interested in, or at least curious about,
brand new methods of diagnosis and treatment?

None of the significance of Dr. Haché's stumbling and
fumbling was lost on Chapdelaine, who, in cross-examination,
arose to rub salt into the now-open wounds of his testimony.
Taking up the question not of a blood, but of a urine, analysis also included in Langlais's medical file, as performed by
Naessens at his microscope, he had the doctor admit, once
again, "I can't understand the way all this is reported, or what
it means. As I said before, I just don't understand what this
examination is all about."

The hapless Haché was unrelentingly drawn further into the embarrassment of his lack of understanding when he was asked by Chapdelaine what he thought of Naessens's method of centrifuging urine to obtain a residue for analysis. Implying that such urine residues were never made, even that they could not be made, he finally expostulated, "Well, at least it's not things we do!" The "we" meaning the medical fraternity in its entirety. And, referring to Naessens's report of *mycelia* (fungoid forms) in the urine, Haché, when asked for his comment by Chapdelaine, could only reply, as helplessly as irritatedly, "They are rarely, if ever, seen! Furthermore, what good would it do to make tests that can't help us with the cancer problem?"

The doctor was now clearly out of his "cutting" depth. It was explained to me by Françoise that, in nuances of his testimony, which I had missed, he had tried to assert, quite erroneously, that *epithelial* cells, if found in the urine, could only come from the epithelium of the skin. What he totally ignored was the fact that they could just as well have come from bladder tissues. And asked whether "crystals" could be found in urine, he replied, "No," though Naessens has repeatedly found them there. Even worse, he equated "albumins" to "proteins," an error of vast proportions, especially with reference to Naessens's unique diagnostics, in that, if found in urine by a special test to prove their presence, they constitute an extremely ominous pathological sign.

It appeared to me that the jurors were not focusing on all this technical discussion. It was as if, to them, the attorney and the doctor were having a private conversation to which they were not privy. Some of them were staring at the ceiling, others at the floor, and one, nodding, was about to doze off, until the stentorian voice of the prosecutor awoke him with a start. Melançon's interruption was to admonish the doctor not to talk just to Chapdelaine, as if in private, but to squarely face and address the jury itself.

Chapdelaine was winding up his cross-examination. "So, doctor," he asked in his ever-quiet manner, "somatids are not familiar to you." He was clearly "rubbing it in" now, making sure that the jury would grasp at least some idea of the doctor's almost complete ignorance of Naessens's methods.

"Well . . . " the surgeon groped again, "there may be some things that could be brought out in blood tests that are not widely known . . . but we don't bother with them."

Chapdelaine: (just short of sarcastically): Could we be having *semantic* problems here?

Haché: Well . . . somatids . . . as I said . . . I seem to recall . . . in a book . . . but we don't use the word *hématie,* * at least not in English, or *asci,* or *levurid.* . . . If a levurid infection in the blood is actually possible, it would take a special exam to detect it."

And, with that, it being 4:30 P.M., court was adjourned by Judge Péloquin, who wished the jury a relaxing weekend.

When the court broke up for the weekend recess, I was able to get an hour of the Naessenses' time, a hard thing to do, given the almost inconceivable pressure they were under. At the Rue Fontaine house, the phone had been literally "ringing off the hook" every few minutes during the several weeks of preparations for the trial, as it kept on ringing even as the trial was in progress.

The scene was unimaginable! Cancer and AIDS victims calling from Québec and from the United States, calls from sufferers who needed no attendance at any medical school to know that the whole orthodox medicine system might send them to their graves, after having preliminarily reached into their pockets, or into the tills of their medical insurance companies, for the average fifty thousand dollars it is estimated

---

*French for "red blood cell."

that a cancer patient must spend on fruitless treatments before his, or her, eventual demise. Well-wishers, advice givers, supplicants, press representatives, and the merely curious—all constantly ringing in on their Rock Forest phone.

And, that weekend, they had almost round-the-clock meetings with Conrad Chapdelaine, their attorney, who, on Saturday came over at noon to stay on until ten o'clock in the evening in order to "get up to speed" on the "ins and outs" of the laboratory work that Naessens had elaborated over four decades, to look into the microscope for the first time, and watch the incredible film made at that instrument that reveals a whole new microscopic world in the blood.

As Françoise put it to me, "Conrad has to know more, much more about what he's defending! When Dr. Haché referred to "fresh blood," he didn't really appreciate what that meant!" At the same time, tit-for-tat, the Naessens had to take their own time with their loyal attorney, and friend, to understand and develop more knowledge of the overall jurisprudential strategy he was preparing.

The behind-the-scenes aspects of what was happening were fascinating to me, much more so than the "formalities" of the courtroom. Françoise took time to explain to me, as she did to her husband's lawyer, more about the mycelial infection that had come up that afternoon, in court. When attacked by fungilike forms, a patient becomes ill enough to exhibit septicemia (a bacteria-induced infection of the blood). This state is detectable only by culturing fresh blood in a medium, in vitro.

The main point was that Haché, as well as most doctors, are wholly unaware that these mycelia are forms in the somatid cycle that have evolved *in* the blood itself, that is, *within* the body. If they *do* see them in the blood, in a "knee-jerk" reaction based on the Pasteurian dogma, they conclude that, if they produce serious states of fever or infection, they must have come from *somewhere outside* the body.

In answer to my probing him about what he would be discussing with Chapdelaine, Naessens told me, "Look! [It's "Hear!"—*Écoutez!*—in French; up to now, I've forgotten to note that Naessens, though he can read some of the language, speaks very little, if any, English] I want Conrad to understand many things that neither he, nor prosecutor Melançon, nor, for that matter, Dr. Haché understood yesterday. So that he can take Haché 'over the jumps' with respect to what he had to say about Madame Langlais's condition. Several times he mentioned Langlais was in an extremely advanced stage of cancer . . . that the ganglion under her armpit had a ninety-nine percent chance of being cancerous. That has to be contrasted with his statement that thirty-five percent of patients, believed curable by orthodox means, have no 'metastases at distance.'"

"If he can be made to admit to the jury that she indeed *had* metastases," Françoise chimed in, "then its members will, or may, understand that there was absolutely *no question* of her having any so-called thirty-five percent survival chance! Chapdelaine will try . . . must be able . . . to show that her visit to us, at what for her was the eleventh hour, in no way retarded, or blocked, any cure."

The Naessenses also told me, with both irony and humor, that, on the day after the trial had begun, their doorbell had rung. On the stoop stood a regional police detective who, handing Naessens his calling card, respectfully requested, almost begged, the biologist to get in contact with one of his colleague's relatives and tell her how, and where, she could be treated for her cancerous condition with 714-X. So, while the whole of the Québec legal system was doing its best to send Naessens to prison for life, one of its representatives was pleading for a cure that the Crown prosecutor, at the trial, was trying to uphold as phony!

The trial entered its second day. The judge and the jury walked in to take their places. "The court is in session . . . please be seated!" intoned the bailiff.

Les jurés, "those sworn (in)," as they are known in French in the plural, from which the collective noun *jury* is derived, looked fresher and more sprightly now that they had rested over the weekend.

Dr. Haché himself reappeared as immaculately tailored as he had been the previous Friday. Naessens, too, was dressed immaculately. He appeared cool and calm, but, for all this external projection, I knew what he was going through. His inner state was betrayed by an occasional "tic" that caused his right eye to flutter about once every three minutes, a tic that I had never seen before in all the ten years I had known him. The frequency of the tic's fluttering would increase. By the end of the trial, it would climb to once a minute, or more.

The ever-suave Judge Péloquin said, "Bonjour Docteur!" The doctor returned the greeting: "Bonjour, Monsieur le Juge!"

Defense attorney Chapdelaine got right down to business. He took the surgeon back to his meeting with Madame Langlais and, asking him with pointed directness whether her cancer state was not fairly "advanced," received Haché's somewhat equivocal answer: "Yes . . . *provisionally.*"

For what seemed an interminably long time, the two professionals, one in law, the other in medicine, discussed the various tests that have been developed to rate the degree of progress in a cancer condition. One of them is the "TMN exam," which evaluates the degree to which *tumors, metastases*, and *nodes* (or ganglia) have developed or become affected. It would only be a tedium for readers to go into all the details.

What Chapdelaine was, of course, continuing to try to establish was that Madame Langlais did indeed have a case of *extremely* advanced cancer plus metastases, which had brought her virtually to death's door even before she decided to give up the horrors of usual treatment and seek an alternative. He went on pressing the doctor: "Did the patient, in fact, have breast cancer that had developed to the point where it had affected the lymph ganglia?"

Haché replied, *"Unequivocally!"* Right at that point, it seemed that Chapdelaine's careful line of questioning was paying large dividends. To consolidate them, he pushed further, taking up a classification of cancer cell types that, depending on whether they are "differentiated," "moderately differentiated," or "nondifferentiated," can have rates of development ranging from slower to much faster, and thus be connected to a prognosis, as far as survival of a cancer patient is concerned, ranging from more to much less hopeful. It was obvious that the attorney for the defense had spent a lot of time on his medical and cancerological homework.

The sought-for consolidation seemed to take shape when another, partially equivocal, statement was forced out of the doctor to the effect that, in cases of breast cancer with metastases, one could be talking of a survival time of only months or even weeks for the patient. "But," added Haché, "I really didn't know whether she actually had metastases associated with 'nondifferentiated' cancer cells, or not."

Chapdelaine was "almost home" in his attempt to convince the jury that Madame Langlais in fact had not the slightest chance of recovery when she decided to take the 714-X treatment. As we shall presently see, the trip "all the way home" was made when he cross-examined the next prosecution witness, a pathologist who had performed an autopsy on the patient after her death.

Though this synopsis may suggest that the facts in the testimony were disclosed in a perfectly logical and sequential manner, such was assuredly not the case. For the prosecutor, who had obviously not done the kind of medical homework as his confrere, seemed, in his own questioning, to wander far from what would provide the proof he was seeking and to meander from one topic to another as if on a "fishing expedition" with no adequate "lure" on his line.

The spotlight was next put by the prosecution on Naessens's product, 714-X. What transpired in court at this point is set down, partially in paraphrase, not so much to transcribe what was actually said, but to show how its content illustrates, once again, the enormous gap—virtually an abyss—between two completely different medical philosophies.

Because what was discussed concerned various "points of law," and especially whether certain testimony would be judged "admissible" or not, the jury, at this point, was dismissed under what is known as *Voir Dire*.

After the jury members departed the courtroom and Haché was asked by Melançon what he knew about Naessens's product, Judge Péloquin broke in, "Hasn't the doctor already said that he didn't know much about it?" To which Haché confessed, "I was a bit vague on the matter."

So that readers can appreciate the substance of the discussion of the "matter," a very important one indeed, not only for the determination of Naessens's juridical fate, but also for the potential application of his product in the broadest medical sphere, part of the repartee among the four participants—judge, surgeon, and the two attorneys—is set down, almost verbatim, from my notes.

Judge: But you said, didn't you, that you did not use it?

Prosecutor (interrupting): Does *any* doctor use it?

Defense: He has said he doesn't know anything about the product, so . . . if he doesn't know, then he doesn't use it. Do you use anything with regard to intralymphatic injection?

Haché (hesitating now): Well, you see . . . I'm not an oncologist . . . or a specialist in medical treatment . . . but through teamwork . . . I learn about . . .

The testimony continued on, with Haché, now clearly on the defensive and unsure of himself as to how to grapple with the problem of "intralymphatic injection," which, up to that moment, had certainly never crossed his path.

Defense: If Dr. Haché says he doesn't know anything about the 714-X product, then why does the prosecutor keep raising the question?

Judge: It seems to me there's another aspect to all this. The doctor is obviously not a specialist in the fabrication, or the assessment of the efficacy, of medicinals. The central question being posed him is whether he, or his colleagues, have *used* the product. I think *he himself* can reply to that, but *not* speak for the medical corps as a whole!

Haché: Well, we, in the medical profession, are aware of what is used, or not, in treatment.

Judge: I think, Maître Chapdelaine, the product may have been used . . . but I also think this question can fairly be asked of the doctor before the jury, if only to let the jury know what *he* knows.

Defense: As long as it doesn't lead the jury into error. Doctor! Did you say the product is used, or useful, or either, or both? How are you capable of asserting that it is *not* useful, if you haven't really looked into the matter in depth?

Haché (slightly irritated): I said it *wasn't* used and *isn't* useful. Look here! Breast cancer is a *very important social problem!* And the hunt is on for a product, any product, that can solve it. But the hunters must be "guided" properly! We must find ways to alter the chemistry of certain products in a given direction, to make them more effective. Such products must have *recognized* properties! You just don't snatch at straws! You don't go putting square pegs into round holes!

Though he did not go so far as to elaborate it, Haché's implication was certainly that 714-X could be nothing but a "square peg." And this alone certainly relates to a general attitude — as noted by Walter Clifford at the second press conference in Sherbrooke — that only research that "toes" an orthodox "line" is acceptable in mainstream medicine. It is also connected to what can be called the "NIH Syndrome," which has nothing to do with the United States' National Institutes of Health (also called NIH) in Washington, D.C., but to the slogan "Not Invented Here," though assuredly a connection between the two identical acronyms might be made.

The attitude was recently most clearly illustrated by the words of the director of one of France's (it could have been any other country's) largest pharmaceutical firms specializing in anticancer products that are made with the unique goal of attacking and killing cancer cells in the body, that is, so-called "chemotherapeutic" products. Those words were addressed to Mirko Beljanski, a Docteur-ès-Sciences, and a researcher for over thirty years at both the famous Institut Pasteur in Paris and at the equally well-known CNRS (Centre National de la Recherche Scientifique), through which scientific inquiry is coordinated in dozens of laboratories all over France. Beljanski, and his wife, Monique, have, over the same thirty years, developed a holistic approach to curing cancer and AIDS that is as startlingly effective as that of Gaston Naessens, who told me that he believes that the couple's methods could most successfully and beneficially be combined with his own. When seeking the industrialist's help to manufacture and market his product, Beljanski began to describe what he had done, he was coldly cut off by the company director with the words: "Look here, Monsieur, you should clearly understand that if I, with my 120 in-house scientists, haven't found a specific anticancer drug, then it's because it simply doesn't exist!" ("Voyons, Monsieur, vous devez bien comprendre que si moi, avec mes 120 chercheurs, je n'ai pas trouvé d'anti-cancéreux spécifiques, c'est bien que ça n'existe pas!")*

The courtroom conversation continued:

*From the Beljanskis' recently published book: *La Santé Confisquée* (Health Confiscated) (France: CIE-12, 1989).

Defense: But this is the very first time you've been confronted with this product?

Haché: Yes.

Defense: So you don't really know what it is, or for that matter, much about it. . . . I mean . . . have you done any analyses on it, or the like?

Haché: No.

Defense: Well, I realize that's not your professional duty.

Haché: Exactly!

Defense: So, as you speak, you are basically relying on what's printed on the label. Have you ever done any reading about the content of the product?

Haché: I've read a few things about camphor.

Defense: But not about camphorminium chloride? You did say, didn't you, that you know of no physicians who have used this product?

Haché: That's right.

Defense: What about Dr. Piers, in Belgium? Dr. Fabre, in France? Drs. Brown and Short, in the United States?

Haché (a little amazed): Are they M.D.s?

Defense: Yes. Sure! And they'll be here to testify at this trial!

Haché: Well, you know there are always a few doctors who do certain things at the margin.

Defense: You consider them "marginal"?

Haché: Yes, marginal, because one should stick to products that have been *tested*, products recognized by the medical profession. Not stuff that's never been heard of! If something's *not known to a large majority, then, by definition, it's not known!*

No statement by a ranking member of the medical profession more clearly reveals the appalling, and helpless, situation that "frontier scientists" such as Gaston Naessens, or the Beljanskis, are forced to occupy. What could easily have been asked of Dr. Haché at this point would be the question: How on earth does anything new *get* known, if it's becoming known runs afoul of the "NIH Syndrome" and the pharmaceutical lobbies, or the governmental licensing mechanisms, that support it?

To try to understand this anomaly, let us digress, for a moment, to read a passage taken from an article entitled "The Quest of the Frontier Scientist," written by physicist Beverly Rubik, Ph.D., director of the Center for Frontier Sciences at Temple University in Philadelphia, which was published in the November/December 1989 issue of *Creation* magazine. Rubik writes:

> Perhaps the greatest obstacle that frontier scientists are unprepared for but inevitably face is *political*—the tendency for human systems to resist change, to resist the impact of new discoveries, especially those that challenge the status quo of the scientific establishment . . . .
>
> . . . "Science" has become institutionalized and is largely regulated by an establishment community that governs and maintains itself. . . . In recent times there has been a narrowing of perspectives resulting in a growing dogmatism, a dogmatic scientism. There is arrogance bordering on worship of contemporary scientific concepts and models . . . taught in our schools in a deadening way which only serves to perpetuate the dogma. . . .
>
> Strangely, the contemporary scientific establishment has taken on the behavior of one of its early oppressors: the church. Priests in white lab coats work in glass-and-steel cathedral-like laboratories, under the rule of bishops and cardinals who maintain orthodoxy through mainstream *"peer review."*

Impressed by this article, which was sent to me as Gaston Naessens's trial was drawing to a close, impressed because

of its pointed *relevancy* to Naessens's situation, I wrote back
to Beverly Rubik to ask a question also relevant to this discussion, namely: *"Peer Review:* How can so-called *peers* be called
on to assess a new invention when they themselves, or at least
the overwhelming majority of them, have *never invented* anything? If they haven't invented anything, in what sense, then,
are they 'peers?'"* For, it seems to me that the true "peer" of an
inventor such as Naessens is someone who has been equally
inventive, not some governmental or private laboratory drone
whose "peerage" is based merely on academic equality.

Everything, in the above digression, was running through
my mind as the conversation in court proceeded:

Defense: So Naessens's product, then, can't be of any importance?

Haché: Well . . . of minor importance.

Defense: It will only become important when a "majority" adopt it?

Haché (again somewhat irritated): Look, there are researchers everywhere trying to seek out new products!

Defense: So you say it's not important!

Haché: Because it may not be in any way applicable!

Defense: Of no interest to you?

Haché: Not really. You see when something really worthwhile is found . . . it's *put to use!*

Defense: When it's officially accepted?

Haché: I've already said that not everything in medicine
that's "discovered" is of importance. Do you know that I've
met doctors in Québec who treat their patients with *pendulums!** You've got to realize that only certain things are really
important!

---

*For information on pendulums, or medical dowsing, see my book
The Divining Hand (*La Main Divinatoire*) (New York: E. P. Dut-
ton, 1979; Paris: Éditions Robert Laffont, 1981).

Defense: Then you have never been involved in research into *experimental* products?

Haché: Only outside my specialty.

Defense: Which is basically surgery?

Haché: Yes, but colleagues who perform the treatments on our patients following surgery . . . give us reports.

Defense: But you, *yourself,* have never become deeply involved in the problem of the assessment of therapeutic products?

Haché: No.

And with that, Doctor Lorenzo Haché, having completed his testimony, repeated most of it over again for the jury, left the stand, the courtroom, and the Palais de Justice, and went home.

Chapter 6
Let No Stone Be Unturned

Innovators are rarely received with joy, and established authorities launch into condemnation of newer truths, for . . . at every crossroads to the future there are a thousand self-appointed guardians of the past.
Betty MacQuitty, *Victory Over Pain:*
Morton's Discovery of Anesthesia

Following Dr. Haché's departure, the next witness called by the prosecution was Dr. Jean-Claude Boivin—the pathologist already mentioned—who had performed an autopsy to show that Madame Langlais's tumor, at the time of her death, had grown to a huge 13–14 centimeters in diameter and that the cancer had metastasized to her liver, lungs, and bone marrow. All of which basically confirmed that she indeed had been affected with cancer impossible to cure by orthodox means long before consulting Naessens.

The following two days were given over to testimonies by the patient's husband, Marcel Langlais, her daughter, and her son-in-law. What the prosecution tried to establish, out of the mouths of these witnesses, was additional proof that Naessens had, in fact, contributed to killing their wife, mother, and mother-in-law. The testimonies went on all day long and, in Langlais's case, ended with his staring loathingly at Gaston Naessens and, with almost a sob rising to a crescendo of emotion, blurting out: "My wife's last words were 'On nous a menti et on nous a trahis!'" (We have been lied to and we have been betrayed), a statement that made the headlines, the next day, in three Québec newspapers.

What the jury did *not* know, during Langlais's protracted testimony, was that his daughter, Marie-France, and his son-in-law, George Kopp, a hospital technician, were close friends of a French-born businessman, Robert Sisso, who, together with his wife, Michèle, had long been friends of the Naessenses.

When Madame Langlais fell ill, the Sissos had pleaded with Naessens to help her. That she was a particularly intimate friend of the couple was illustrated by the fact that the second series of 714-X treatments she received were injected into her by Michèle herself, who had stated to Françoise Naessens, "Even when Madame Langlais finally was forced into hospital, she told her daughter that she still held Naessens in high regard! Furthermore, it was a fact that George Kopp had told Robert Sisso that his mother-in-law, were she still alive, would never have permitted her daughter to denounce Naessens to the Medical Corporation as she actually had done after her mother's death."

Since the jury was unaware of all these facts, the main effect of the Langlais testimony, from the point of view of the defense attorney, was his being able to raise a doubt in cross-examination, in the minds of the jurors. In so doing, Chapdelaine did not dispute the fact that Madame Langlais had received treatment by Naessens but, instead, did his best to show that the cancer victim had consistently refused conventional treatment and deliberately opted for the 714-X injections of her own volition.

As I have stated earlier, the testimony by the Langlais trio, as it was drawn from them by prosecution questions, came out, just as it did for those of preceding witnesses, not in any orderly or logical fashion, but piecemeal and "helter-skelter." I suffered for the jury, as I attempted to follow the several descriptions of what exactly happened in the meetings at the Naessenses' Rock Forest house and write down notes upon them.

One thing should certainly be added concerning the prosecution's apparent misjudgment in calling as one of its witnesses Roland Caty, who, as we remember, was one of the first patients to treat himself, while in Africa, with 714-X, and thus recover from his prostate cancer after having been threatened with an operation to cut off his penis and his testicles. Caty, who had become involved with injecting Madame Langlais after she returned to Montréal, was questioned by Melançon to try to establish certain negative aspects of her treatment. Little did the prosecutor suspect that, instead of mainly testifying against Naessens as he had hoped, Caty would swing round in court to rebound against Melançon and to provide all details of how he owed his life to a self-taught biologist! The jury was thus able to listen to the entire saga of his recovery.

While speaking of Caty, it is also fitting to bring up another prosecution witness who, in his way, also boomeranged. The man in question was Yugoslavian-born Stephen Zalac, a naturopath of almost military bearing, who was called in connection with charges of "bodily harm" and "fraud" caused to a second patient implicated in the charges against Naessens. In that same connection, Zalac had already paid a heavy fine for "illegal practice of medicine" and, consequently, was immune from further prosecution. What Melançon wanted to prove, through Zalac's testimony, was "complicity" between the naturopath and Gaston Naessens with respect to the counts of bodily harm and fraud.

It was revealed that Zalac had, for years, been a member of the board of directors of the McNaughton Foundation, founded by a Canadian general, Andrew McNaughton, which has since moved from Québec to California. The objectives of the foundation have long been the promotion of "frontier" research in medicine and other sciences. As a therapist, Zalac had "been around." Having met Naessens and his wife over twenty years ago, and having later experimented with the 714-X product in Mexico at the clinic of Dr. Alejandro Andrade, president of the Medical Society of the State of Vera Cruz, he has worked with doctors in Europe and the United States on aspects of "alternative" medicine for many years.

Zalac got the chance to inform the jury that, despite the fact that Québec physicians are *poursuivis* (a French "umbrella" word that can mean "investigate," "make a case against," "prosecute," and several other things) if they have anything to do with naturopaths, he had nevertheless been cooperating closely with several who had had the courage to do so.

Delivering his testimony in a forthright, matter-of-fact manner, in a voice emanating nothing but honesty and confidence, Zalac described his visits to Rock Forest on behalf of the patient concerned as being necessary for the sole purpose of getting the blood and urine exams needed for assessing at what stage the somatid cycle in the body had progressed. These tests he had then compared with standard blood tests made in regular labs through the cooperation of his doctor associates.

With the jury dismissed under another *Voir Dire* session, the next witness, called by the prosecution to give data on the Naessens-MacDonald-Stewart connection, was Guy Ducharme, a foundation employee. Ducharme stated that David Stewart, who unexpectedly died in hospital after returning from a trip to Switzerland in 1984, had, in the tradition of his forebears, endowed chairs at several Montréal institutions of higher learning, including the world-famous McGill University.

According to Ducharme, one of Stewart's chief beliefs was that people should be rated not for the academic honors they had won, or for the positions they held in society or the professional sphere, but mainly for their inherent abilities, individual capacities, and their strength of character—which could explain a lot about why he had come to back Naessens.

Stewart had become interested in the whole problem of cancer in his youth, when a dear friend had died of the disease while only in his forties. In the early 1970s, he set up two schools for cytology (study of normal and cancerous cells), one at McGill University, the other at the wholly Francophone Université de Montréal.

At this point, the prosecutor haughtily interrupted with a question: "What I don't understand at all is why a supporter of serious cancer research got involved with Naessens. Can you enlighten me?" This obvious put-down of Naessens was lost neither on many people in the audience nor, perhaps, on several members of the jury.

Returning to what amounted to Stewart's "private war" on cancer, Ducharme said it had been declared before, in fact, long before, he had met the biologist. Part of the motivation for it had come from Stewart's mother, a nurse in her own right. "Monsieur David Stewart," stressed Ducharme, "repeatedly cited a formula, or motto, to everyone around him, especially those involved in orthodox cancer research: 'Let no stone be unturned in the search for truth, or the cure for cancer!'" Its corollary, of course, was that, if orthodox medicine could not come up with a cure, after the expenditure of billions of dollars worldwide, then that cure would have to be found "somewhere . . . anywhere . . . else."

By leading Ducharme to review a series of grants made by his foundation to support academic research on Naessens's "science," Melançon's main aim was to demonstrate that though Stewart had spent over $1,500,000 to verify the effectiveness of Naessens's methods over more than fifteen years, the foundation had only negative results to show for it. But, as we shall see, the prosecutor was careful to reveal only the reverse of that coin while keeping its obverse concealed.

First among these efforts was a three-year program undertaken at the Medical Centre of McMaster University in Hamilton, Ontario, which ran from 1972 to 1975, at a cost of $200,000 a year. That this project, like others that followed it, could be characterized as having certain "Byzantine" aspects may be deduced from what follows.

Even before calling Ducharme, Melançon had put on the stand Peter Dent, M.D., chairman of McMaster University's Pediatrics Department, who also bore the imposing title "consultant in immunology to the Ontario Cancer Foundation," a position one would have thought would make him particularly interested in Naessens's research. During his negative, at times hostilely negative, testimony, Dent had trouble remembering some of the things that had transpired in connection with the research project. And some of the things he did say could easily be interpreted as revealing how the investigations funded by David Stewart had often been shoddily or mistakenly performed.

As a prime example of this, one can cite Dent's reference to his use of one of Naessens's "anticancer" preparations, then called ISO-412, later called Kelectomine. When asked by Chapdelaine, under cross-examination, whether, in fact, this product had been developed, not as a cancer-countering agent, but as a nonsurgical means of amputation, Dent somewhat confusedly replied, *"Probably* correct!" Something strange was going on.

Kelectomine, a word fashioned from Greek roots meaning to "sever beyond," had, in fact, been developed by Naessens over the years 1965–1966, and a long film had been made on its use on rats. When injected into a section of one of the limbs of a rat—or any other mammal—it almost miraculously causes that section, and the whole portion of the limb below it, painlessly and antiseptically to drop off the body within about three days. If, for example, a whole limb—an arm or a leg—requires amputation, the product is accordingly injected into the upper arm or the thigh such that the limb falls off, either at the shoulder or the hip joint. If injected lower down the limb, say, in the lower arm, or the calf, what falls off is that portion of the leg below the knee joint, or the arm below the elbow. This is because the product cannot affect any part of the limb above the next joint below which it is injected due to the fact that it cannot penetrate, or pass through, a membrane, located in each mammalian body joint, known as a perimysium.

When, in the late 1970s, during one of my earlier visits to Rock Forest, I learned of Kelectomine's remarkable properties and saw its effect on rats, I prevailed on a friend, Boston biochemist Boguslaw Lipinski, Ph.D., D.Sc., to travel to Naessens's lab to check it out. Lipinski was impressed with the documented cancer-curative properties of 714-X, but, when told of the amputative properties of Kelectomine, he was more than baffled. As he later informed me, "When Naessens told me what I thought was a 'fairy story,' I began to have serious doubts about the whole of his work!"

Sensing Lipinski's disbelief, Naessens smilingly gave the biochemist two vials of Kelectomine and suggested that, when he was back in his lab in a Boston hospital, he inject their contents into the thighs of two rats to see what might happen. And that is exactly what Lipinsky did, in the dead of night, so that no one would know what he was doing. And just as Naessens told him they would, within three days one of each rat's hind legs detached from its body so painlessly that the rats themselves, throughout the amputative process, continued their normal behavior, eating, drinking, moving about, and even copulating.

Lipinski was stunned by the implication that so simple a method could provide, as an alternative to expensive surgical cutting, as radical an approach to painless amputation as had been offered by anesthesia in the nineteenth century, following a long history of excruciatingly painful amputations on conscious human beings.

Given that background, none of which was known to the jury, judge, the press, or most of the spectators, it was my turn to become stunned when I heard cancer researcher Dent reply to Chapdelaine's question with the answer: "*Probably* correct!" If the good doctor was not sure about the purpose of a product he was using, then what had been going on in Hamilton in the mid-1970s? Could it have possibly been that Dent, who took little trouble to consult with Naessens himself about anything, had been improperly briefed as to the properties, and proper use, of various products?

Whatever the case, Chapdelaine, sticking to his course, was trying to show, with his questions to Dent, that a product with which McMaster was at the time experimenting bore no relation at all to 714-X, the one used in connection with the two patients at issue in the trial, a product considered by the prosecution to be phony and the *only* one ever developed by Naessens. He stated to the judge that Dent, incapable of identifying the products, singly, or one from another, was "putting apples and carrots in the same hamper."

As he had of Dr. Haché, Chapdelaine also asked Dent what he knew about somatids and whether he had ever seen them. This line of questioning produced a series of incoherent answers, indicating that the professor either knew very little or, if he did, was not about to admit it. The exchange led in no particular direction, in fact just went "round and round."

Asked, finally, if McMaster had ever published any results for the MacDonald-Stewart Foundation, Dent curtly said, "No!" Asked why not, he replied, "Because we felt it wasn't *bona fide* science!"

To which, Chapdelaine queried: "How can you say that?"

And Dent answered, "Because most of the observations made by Naessens were based on error, or were already known to the scientific community."

"Is that your opinion?" queried Chapdelaine.

"Yes!" replied Dent.

Dent's testimony seemed to have left the judge, the press table members, the spectators, and certainly myself completely "in the dark" as to the true nature and substance of its details.

Trying to sort some of this out, Judge Péloquin, rightly analyzing the situation, said, "The work done at the time, by Dent and his colleagues, certainly can't be compared to the work done since, which goes all the way up to 1989." This statement was for the benefit of the prosecutor. And it also seemed partially to chide him for presenting a witness whose statements were irrelevant to the trial and thus inadmissible for the jury.

So challenged, the prosecutor, in a partial retreat, allowed, "I'll admit only that in the 1970s' work McMaster University was unsuccessful." This statement immediately provoked a protest from the defense: "That's a very dangerous line. . . . He's trying to establish that, since 1972, it's *all the same product.* He's not at all interested in laying bare what all the various products were, or are, or how they are used . . . just as if they were all the same!"

Never altering the half smile that seemed permanently to crease his face, Judge Péloquin said quietly, "Early work done at McMaster University turned out negative." Then, directly to Melançon: "I won't let you go further on that! There was no comparison made on the use of various products. I agree with Maître Chapdelaine on that!"

It was becoming obvious that, if a courtroom may at times not be a place where truth is easily revealed, it certainly also was no venue to shed light on scientific research.

Chapter 7
The Dam of Dogma

Peer review is widely seen as the modern touchstone of truth. Scientists are roundly drubbed if they bypass it and "go public" with their research. . . . The first limitation of peer review is that nobody can say quite what it is. . . . A more pernicious danger is that peer review may reject the important work. As Charles W. McCutchen, a physicist at the National Institutes of Health, has put it, peers on the panel reviewing a grant applicant "profit by his success in drawing money into their collective field, and by his failure to do revolutionary research that would lower their own ranking in the profession. It is in their interest to approve expensive, pedestrian proposals."

Jonathan Schlefer, Editorial,
Technology Review, October 1990

To truly understand what transpired at the McMaster University Medical Centre, in all its torturous convolutions, one must take into account a complex chain of events in a drama the panoply of which was never brought out in court, mainly because attorney Chapdelaine felt that its inclusion would be spurious to his overall strategy.

Some of that history is summarized here, in barest outline, so that readers can understand what was taking place both behind the scenes and in the "hearts and minds" of certain members of the dramatis personae, which could easily have come from the pen of a scientific Machiavelli.

The history began on 28 March 1972, when the Naessenses made an initial visit to Hamilton, where they met with Dent and his colleagues, including a bright, young, and in-

quisitive assistant professor of pathology and surgery named
Daniel Y. E. Perey. In his midthirties, Perey, who had done
his graduate work in both Canada and the United States, realized, from the very outset, that, from what the Naessenses
had told the McMaster group, David Stewart was onto "something big."

Volunteering to take charge of the foundation-funded
investigation, Perey understood that what was required of
him was no narrow study but an in-depth "look-see" at the
broadest possible spectrum of Naessens's findings, the entire
sweep of his microscopic discoveries, or, to cite the foundation document that collectively characterized them: *Nu* biology, the *Nu* literally representing the Greek letter "N," for
Naessens, and vocally equivalent to the English word "new."

To begin his awesome assignment, Perey spent eleven
days in April working with Naessens in his Rock Forest
laboratory, where, as he later wrote, "I entered a veritable
ocean of new research!" The assignment was a pleasant one
on several counts, not the least of which, as he told Françoise Naessens, was the perquisite of being able to dine in
restaurants offering "La bonne bouffe française," so wholly
lacking in Hamilton, Ontario.

During long conversations in French with Naessens,
the bilingual Perey was introduced, via the microscope, to
the amazing cloud of somatids that one can see shimmering in
the blood, looking, for all the world, like "snow" on a television
screen, a cloud that Perey likened to a "dust storm."

Over the succeeding months, Perey would return to Rock
Forest several times more. On 28 April 1972, the now-excited
Perey brought Dent and another McMaster Medical Centre
colleague, Dr. John Bienenstock, to Rock Forest, where the
whole day was given over, in an initial extensive briefing of
the newcomers, to consultations and conversations with Naessens about the direction Perey would take in further research.

Dent, however, perhaps skeptical of and annoyed by a

whole philosophy heretical to his medical learning, seemed far less impressed than Perey, for, less than a week later, as his own first "research effort," he wrote to the National Cancer Institute of Canada to ask for its evaluation of the biologist and his work.

In reply, the institute sent Dent a single page from a much longer report, "Unproven Methods of Cancer Treatment," compiled by its "sister," or "mother," organization, the American Cancer Society, for circulation to fifty-eight of its divisions. Entitled "Naessens's Serum or Anablast," the single page, after referring in some detail to the French investigation that had purportedly determined the product's so-called worthlessness, ended abruptly with the observation that Naessens had been found guilty of illegal medical practice in his home country and heavily fined.

That any fair investigation of the lifelong research of any man could *begin* by dredging up dirt that had been cast on him abroad certainly did not seem to offer much foundation for Naessens's hope that he would find any "open-mindedness" toward his discoveries on the part of ranking Canadian doctors that had been desperately lacking in their French counterparts. In fact, here was one of them relying, for his own evaluation, on a brief report issued by an investigative body long known to have played the chief role of stamping out any alternative cancer cures unapproved by the cancer establishment.

Whatever Dent's private motivations, the investigations David Stewart was commissioning remained, for a time at least, under Perey's and not Dent's aegis. Excited by his view of a microbiological "continent" as new to his eyes, in 1972, as the "West Indies" had been to Christopher Columbus's in 1492, Perey, after close observation of every one of the forms in the somatid cycle proliferating, even as he watched, strongly recommended to Stewart that his foundation purchase equipment that would allow Naessens to make moving pictures— as well as time-lapse still photos—of all these wonders.

This equipment was supplied through the offices of Wild Leitz, the well-known German optical company, whose Montréal branch's chief executive officer, Leonard LeBel, was to become deeply impressed with the potential of Naessens's microscope. In a letter of 28 May 1976, LeBel wrote to Naessens: "I personally believe your discoveries must become much better known to the scientific world and promoted as soon as possible for the well-being of our population." And in a second letter, dated 25 October 1977:

> It is with pride that I am transmitting to Monsieur Dieter Heid, Canadian General Manager of our Division of Microscopy, your invitation to view, and to have a look through, the Naessens microscope, one of the great advantages of which can be easily seen to be the guarantee of a higher resolution at magnifications at least double those available with optical solutions presently in use.

Perey, of course, was not interested in *how* the magnifying instrument worked, *why* its "mathematical constants" had not been deciphered, or *whether* it "obeyed optical laws." It was enough for him to be able to delve microscopically into a new scientific frontier. To try to impart some of his excitement to his McMaster colleagues, Perey arranged for the Naessenses to travel to Hamilton, where they spent three days at the Medical Centre. Before setting forth, they took the trouble to load the microscope into the back seat of Naessens's car, no mean task in that it had to be specially crated so that it would remain absolutely immobile throughout the 950-mile round trip.

At Hamilton, Naessens showed all of the films he had made that revealed the metamorphosis of the somatid into its successive forms and, using noncancerous and cancerous mice supplied by the hospital, got the researchers to see for themselves through his microscope that many of the forms developed only in the sick animals.

The *Nu* biologist also gave an hour-long lecture, translated word by word from the French by Perey, covering every aspect of his discoveries. During this lecture, he told his audience that, with the use of a special dark-field microscope, they would be able to see, if not the somatids themselves, many of the forms into which they proliferated, and thus, even in the absence of his own instrument, be able to perform serious studies on their behavior.

On 22 September 1972, Perey, in a report to David Stewart entitled "What Has Been Done to Date," enthusiastically set down the whole universe of novelties that had come to his attention, and stated that he had been struck almost "dumb" by the somatid cycle and what he called its "tremendous polymorphism" with respect to size, shape, and other characteristics of its forms. Particularly amazing to Perey was the ability of these forms to resist temperatures over the boiling point as well as ultraviolet radiation, procedures commonly used to "sterilize" any material, that is, to kill any microbes existing within it. Part of this same amazement applied to specific mycelial forms, which, because they looked and behaved like common fungi, should, in Perey's view, have been susceptible to, and therefore annihilatable by, fungicidal antibiotics. But, as he reported to Stewart: "In spite of the extremely high doses of such drugs applied to them, the 'bugs' grew happily. They must therefore be considered not only resistant to the killing drugs, but also be quite different from what appear to be their first cousins."

The report contained many other details, one of the most important of which was Perey's having seen, "beyond the shadow of doubt," that whereas "normal bugs," the first three stages of the somatid cycle, had appeared in the blood of "normal" rats unafflicted with cancer, "abnormal bugs," the successive thirteen stages in the cycle, had appeared in the blood of rats that had received transplantable cancer tumors.

Even more striking was Perey's astonishment that, as

he put it, "while each of the separate forms showed some characteristics of organisms well known in standard micro-biology—bacteria, fungi, and viruses—the big difference was that, far from living independently, one from another, they had all seemed to derive from 'one bug.'"

The extent to which Perey had become impressed with what he had seen and studied was made clear in a formal letter he wrote, on 29 September 1972, to Canadian immigration authorities to whom Gaston Naessens had made application for the "landed immigrant" status that would legalize his permanent residence in Québec and open the way to his attaining Canadian citizenship. An "appeals board" before which Perey had testified in June had denied Naessens's petition. Also signed by Perey's colleague Associate Professor of Medicine John Bienenstock, the letter referred to the fact that their scientific investigations of certain "claims" made by the biologist, "highly relevant to the field of biology in general and to cancer in particular," by providing "further insight," had convinced the McMaster researchers that the appeals board should "be made aware of their basic and potential significant implications, and of the desirability of the continued presence of Mr. Naessens in this country."

"At a time," read the concluding paragraph,

when a hundred million dollars have been infused into the field of cancer research in the United States, and with some personal knowledge of the unimaginative approaches toward diagnosis and treatment of this scourge of mankind, we feel that it is the responsibility of anyone, however tenuously connected, to support any attempt to further substantiate an original and imaginative approach. In our opinion, Mr. Naessens is essential for this to occur. The scope and insight which he has brought to this area of research potentially stand to benefit mankind and may be a source of pride to Canada.

The above-cited letter, the only one of its kind ever to be signed by qualified medical researchers, not only won for Naessens the acceptance of his request to become a permanent resident, but seemed to promise the rosiest of horizons as far as the future of his research and its formal acceptance by the medical community was concerned. That such was not the case was evidenced, more than two years later, by another letter Perey was forced to write Naessens, to which was attached a copy of a final, and negative, report sent to the MacDonald-Stewart Foundation.

So what happened in the interim? To try to answer this important question, let us here examine some of the wording in the letter. "Although you might receive this report as a condemnation of your work," wrote Perey, "it is not written with this intention. We have come to different conclusions and interpretations based on the scientific evidence which we gathered, although in many instances we have observed identical or similar phenomena as you have." This conclusion was as much a smoke screen to hide certain "happenings" at McMaster as a clear spotlight on what had actually transpired.

To give readers but an inkling of these happenings, we might offer Françoise's statement that, during a third visit by herself and her husband to McMaster, she had asked Dent whether he and his colleagues had, in fact, succeeded in isolating the somatids in order to see whether, among other things, they contained DNA.

Almost incomprehensibly, Dent only replied, "We did succeed but, unfortunately, we broke the test tube containing the somatid culture!"

While "mysteries," such as the above, were never clarified, a significant change in the McMaster research became crystal clear when, at the end of 1972, Daniel Perey was assigned to "other duties," many of them administratively time-consuming, and responsibility for *Nu* biology passed into the hands of two bacteriological specialists, a husband-

and-wife team of Indian extraction, the Banerjees. It was after their appointment that relations between Naessens and McMaster University began to sour.

In late 1972, Dr. Perey brought the Banerjees to the Rock Forest lab, where the Naessenses were naturally eager to learn whether his replacements would continue to follow the broad investigative trail Perey had already blazed. To their utter astonishment, they were informed by the Banerjees in an arrogant tone that, since *they* were now "in charge," things would be done *"their* way." "Their way" meant that, because of their past research experience as bacteria specialists, they were particularly interested in, and wanted to focus exclusively upon, a bacterial form in the somatid cycle that German researchers had come across as long ago as the 1930s, and investigate whether a claim by the Germans that it had an effect on rheumatism was true or not. Thus, while Perey had set his sight on analyzing a whole checkerboard of problems, the Banerjees, it seemed to the Naessenses, were reducing the scope of their interest to only one of its squares.

Since neither the husband nor the wife spoke a word of French, Françoise, trying to establish some kind of relationship with them more direct than could be achieved through interpreter Perey, asked in English: "But, by working on the problem of *just one bacterium,* you won't be able to achieve Mr. Stewart's goal of proving whether the whole of Monsieur Naessens's discoveries and theory is correct or not, will you?"

The husband's answer was shocking to Françoise's ears: "We are certainly not here to prove whether your husband is 'right' or 'wrong,' Mrs. Naessens! What we are here to do is to discuss a project of interest to *us,* and that concerns solely the bacteria."

So the whole goal, as envisioned by David Stewart, was being thrown out the window. When the Naessenses tried to say so, the Banerjees, ignoring their protest, said they were "offended" by the Naessenses' position concerning their research ideas and "insulted" by their attitude. Since they had been appointed by the foundation to carry on the research, they concluded, they would proceed with that task "exactly as they saw fit," and that was that.

After the Banerjees departed, Gaston and Françoise Naessens dejectedly drove to Montréal with Perey for a conference with David Stewart. At a meeting in his office, Perey valiantly tried to play a mediator's role while Naessens tried to explain to Stewart what the foundation director already knew: that the Banerjees were piloting the ship of his research project not into the port of its planned destination, but, by crazily veering off course, driving it directly onto the rocks. As for David Stewart, an introverted and never assertive man, he merely sat quietly and somewhat remotely, listening to the threesome's comments.

Despite the Naessenses' advice that he stop funding the McMaster project as a waste of money, Stewart elected to continue it, partly because the Banerjees had given up alternate research appointments and he did not want to leave them "high and dry." The decision was a disastrous one, mainly due to the fact that Stewart was unaware of the narrow-mindedness and strong prejudices ingrained in the couple's scientific outlook.

From ongoing correspondence with the foundation, always signed by Perey, it can be seen that the Banerjees never could get rid of their consuming doubt that "events" observed in fresh blood under the microscope actually "represented the appearance of latent organisms normally repressed in the blood circulation of healthy subjects." Like many other observers before them and many to come, they held to belief that the same events had been only artificially induced, due to the "abnormal environment necessary for the observation of such blood." In other words, they were nothing but mistakenly produced *artifacts*.

These conclusions more than justified fears expressed

by Naessens to Perey and Stewart when he first learned what the line of research proposed by the Banerjees was likely to be. In one report to the foundation sent in the middle of July 1973, for instance, Perey, who had hoped to allay those fears in private conversations with Naessens, tried to define their basis: "In essence," he wrote, "this represents the long and extensive acquaintance of Mr. Naessens with *Nu* organisms, shaded at times with personal hypothesis, as opposed to our relatively recent entry into the picture shaded by *our more classical scientific background and dogmas.*" The last seven words of that sentence have been italicized for emphasis, because they imply more, a great deal more, than might be comprehended at first glance. Their implication is that Naessens's findings and theories about the true nature of degenerative disease, and the medically important theoretical conclusions resulting from them, were not acceptable only because, never having entered the precincts of "received knowledge," or accepted *dogma*, they had never been taught, at least not to the Banerjees.

More serious was a final "point of disagreement" to which Perey referred: "For some unknown reasons, the McMaster group has been unable to repeat certain studies which seemingly are routinely successful in Mr. Naessens's hands, making joint studies both in Sherbrooke and at McMaster highly relevant at this stage."* There were, it seemed, "nuances" of technique that the "debutantes" in Hamilton, Ontario, needed to learn from the "master" in Rock Forest.

It is not until one proceeds, in Perey's ongoing correspondence with Stewart, to his letter of 13 December 1973, that one learns exactly what studies the Banerjees had been "unable to repeat."One of these, the doctor noted, was "the recovery of microorganisms from blood cultures of cancer patients and normal individuals." It seemed that the Banerjees were,

---

*The recommended "joint studies" never took place.

in fact, declaring that a simple technique to extract forms from the somatid cycle from the blood was as difficult, or impossible, as Dr. Haché had declared injections into the lymph system to have been.

Perey also tempered his conclusion with a bit of better news: "I am happy to report," he added, "that, after nearly one impossible year for all of us, we are now beginning to observe microorganisms from nearly all of our blood cultures." Did this mean that the technique had been learned? Even if it had, it did not also mean that the need to isolate, and culture, the new microbiological forms was being recognized in all its true significance. For Perey felt constrained to continue: "These bugs have morphological characteristics similar to what Mr. Naessens has described, but I hasten to add that these are so far strictly morphologic characteristics which in no way elucidate their nature." This apparently meant that, because they had never been seen by anyone but Naessens, and were not "in the books," they could therefore not be explained.

A little more positively, Perey continued: "Nevertheless, this initial critical step is most exciting, since we are now in a position to study them and their relationship to disease. Moreover, this adds credibility to the initial observation, and to its originator." In all the darkness, was light beginning to loom at the end of a tunnel?

Perey went on to admit his "frustration" at not being able to explain why it had taken so long for the organisms to "appear." The fact that some of the somatid cycle forms appeared in the blood of both healthy humans and cancer patients, he wrote, "does not negate, even may support, Monsieur Naessens's thesis that all individuals harbor *Nu* organisms, which are held in check during health but somehow escape 'surveillance' in diseased patients. . . . The difficult question remains to determine whether the transformed bugs actually *cause* disease as opposed to being the result of disease, and we should all remain realistic and be prepared for a very difficult struggle."

Perey did not mention that that same "struggle," in addition to being an outward one, objectively connected with scientific research, was also, perhaps mainly, an inward one, subjectively connected with the crying need to overcome prejudices about the origin of disease that went all the way back to the controversy between Pasteur and Béchamp!

"Our excitement," Perey continued somewhat enigmatically, "should be viewed as a first step, strictly speaking, although one cannot deny that subsequent steps might be just as exciting, indeed even more so." From his correspondence, it was clear that Perey was caught between two "stools." On the one hand, he was trying to confirm his early enthusiasm, based on his own experimental work done with Naessens. On the other, he was valiantly attempting to support scientific colleagues in their own conclusions, while recognizing that these conclusions could well have been severely flawed by bias. A key sentence in Perey's letter seems to indicate this recognition: "Indeed, microbiological dogmas are so entrenched in the Banerjees' minds that they do not allow themselves the luxury of challenging them, thereby making each new observation perhaps more difficult but, by necessity, more solid."

Carefully worded as Perey's statement was to avoid more direct confrontation, one might well ask: How on earth can the destruction of "entrenched dogma" be characterized as a "luxury"? Could not the phrase "not allow themselves the luxury of challenging" easily be translated to mean "neither want to use or even to consider a new approach"? And, knowing, in all likelihood, that this was actually the case, Perey, trying to mitigate the suspicion, or to soften it in Stewart's eyes, somewhat weakly concluded: "Regardless of dogmas, I can assure you that both classical, as well as less orthodox, culture methods, approaches, and interpretations will be followed in the future."

Despite this assertion, in a subsequent missive to Stewart, Perey was obviously ceding more ground to the dogmatists' entrenched idea that the novel forms discovered by Naessens, far from being anything new or important in nature, had, indeed, been artificially produced. As the doctor wrote: "Dogma has it that the forms represented are only *artifactual* phenomena, although we failed to document this in electron microscopy." Despite the lack of documentation, the dogma held as rigidly as ever. Even after referring once again, to "artifact," Perey nevertheless could go on to comment: "It is of interest that the strange forms are now seen in at least one blood culture after several months. . . . Should we succeed in 'growing' these forms in secondary cultures, it will be very difficult to maintain that they are red blood cell membranes!" Such a comment suggests that he was still trying to get the Banerjees to overcome their dogma, a task that he obviously could not fulfill.

The power of that dogma was also illustrated to me during an early 1980s' visit to Naessens's laboratory of the chief scientist for a well-known biomedical research institution in Massachusetts. After spending nearly a whole day observing somatid-cycle forms in Naessens's microscope, this man only later, once out of Naessens's presence, declared that everything he had seen in connection with the cycle was artifact. Invited to sign Naessens's guest book, which contains plaudits from many researchers around the world, the chief scientist rudely refused.

How could a *Nu*, or new, science ever prevail in the face of an old one's being unable to give up its prejudice, or even to learn from its mistakes?

The McMaster effort, which had so much promise when overseen by Daniel Perey, finally ended in complete failure. What the Naessenses, as they told me, always hoped was that, with David Stewart's support, an official university team of scientists, capably instructed, and honestly motivated, would be able to replicate the easily performed isolation and culturing of the somatids.

Following that, what the Naessenses wanted determined, with lab equipment and methods more sophisticated than those available to them in Rock Forest, was, first of all, the exact chemical composition of the somatids, to reveal the connection with DNA, a finding that, if confirmed, might be as important to science as the discovery of the nature of DNA itself, reported many years ago in John Watson's scientific thriller *The Double Helix* (New York: Atheneum, 1968).

Second, the Naessenses were looking for help in identifying the growth hormone that proliferates in the blood as a result of the onset of the pathological extension of the normal somatid cycle, to see whether or not it did, in fact, correspond to what Alexis Carrel had named a trephone, as well as in identifying toxins emitted by cancer cells to which they had given the name the "Cocancerogenic K Factor."

Third, the Naessenses were confident that, had the work been correctly performed, their firm conclusion that degenerative diseases, such as cancer, can be prediagnosed long before their clinical signs appear, would have been recognized years ago. That, in turn, together with a recognition of the effectiveness of their treatment, might have by now resulted in a steep drop in new cases of cancer, which each year have grown in numbers.

"I believe," Françoise told me, "that had Dr. Perey been able to continue his direction of the work he commenced in 1972, he would have succeeded in attaining the goals we mapped out, and publication of his results would have gone far to convince a great number of honest scientists and doctors. Most important, the scientific world would have been made aware of the startling breakthroughs achieved by Naessens."

Chapter 8
Someone or Something

If I contracted cancer, I would never go to a standard cancer treatment center. Cancer victims who live far from such centers have a chance.

> Professor Georges Mathé, French cancer specialist, "Scientific Medicine Stymied," *Médecines Nouvelles* (Paris), March 1989

Aghast that the expensive McMaster research, so promising at its inception, had foundered on the shoals of narrow-mindedness, David Stewart was at his wit's end concerning where to find "another stone to turn." Quite unexpectedly, this stone appeared when, one winter day in 1978, Stewart was visited in his office by Dr. Jan Merta de Velehrad, a Czech-born Canadian, who for the past ten years had been his adopted country's "Chief Inspector of Diving," a specially created post to which he won appointment after being selected for it, in competition, from among many international applicants. As "Tsar" of all deep-sea diving activities in Canadian oceans, from the mouth of the St. Lawrence River, to the Queen Charlotte Strait in the Pacific, to the Arctic's Beaufort Sea, Merta holds responsibility for the maintenance of the highest standards of diving techniques and technology, and for the safety of all those practicing one of the world's most hazardous professions. He also possesses a Ph.D. in psychology from Aberdeen University in Scotland.

I had met Jan Merta in 1969, when, after a hair-raising escape from Czechoslovakia, he arrived in Montréal. For the new few years, we met frequently in the gerontology laboratory of Dr. Bernard Grad in the Allan Memorial Institute of Psychiatry attached to McGill University, where Jan was pursuing undergraduate studies in zoology, physiology, and psychology. An inventive genius in his own right, and gifted with exceptional "psychic" talents since childhood, he spent many hours telling me about his life story, which could itself be the subject of an exciting book.

As Grad's assistant, Merta designed a number of fascinating devices and experiments on such novel topics as the influence of magnetic fields on the properties of water and on the learning ability of rats, and on their offspring, affected by the same fields. "Unfortunately, as a result of my intensive study in psychic research, and my demonstrated abilities," he recalled to me, "and my having established a certain international public 'notoriety' in this academically taboo area, I was, for my pains, only branded with the 'Mark of Cain,' so much so that I strongly doubt that, due to my involvement with ESP, any of my other scientific work will ever be accepted in academic circles.

"As a result, I decided to have done with all such pursuits, dear as they were to me, and completely devote myself to something brand new, a 'down-to-earth' activity that turned out to be deep-sea diving and its problems, a field in which, for the last seventeen years, I have made my career. Even if I have never regretted my 'change of direction,' when I look back, on occasion, I sometimes feel sorry for those a priori skeptics who, though they viciously attacked my work, my contributions, and my character, have themselves contributed virtually nothing of significance to new knowledge and to our understanding, and they never will."

When, in 1977, I came face to face with the novelty of Gaston Naessens's work, I was consumed both by excitement and by doubt. So, to allay my initial uncertainty, I called on my scientist friend Jan Merta de Velehrad, who visited Naessens in his lab and was introduced to the research during the whole of a cold December day. At Naessens's recommendation, Jan decided to look up David Stewart, partly because Stewart's wife, Lillian, also had a Czech background.

Though Stewart could not give him an immediate appointment, he told Jan that he would soon be going over to Scotland, where Merta, at the time, was working as director for research and development for Oceaneering International, one of the world's largest underwater engineering firms. In Aberdeen, Merta showed Stewart around many facilities, including a diving hospital, the first of its kind, that he had helped to design and build. During the tour, the pair got to "know each other," and Stewart invited Merta to revisit him in Montréal the next time he crossed the Atlantic.

When they next came face to face in Stewart's office, Merta, intrigued by what he had seen on his repeated visits to Rock Forest, boldly asked Stewart "how in hell" it was that a staunch backer of orthodox medical research had so loyally supported Naessens's work for so many years. "By way of reply," said Merta, in December 1989, "Stewart told me the following story, which I shall repeat from memory.

"While he was still a young man, David Stewart's family had a gardener in its employ who had worked in that position for as long as he, Stewart, could remember. The gardener came down with a severe cough, was hospitalized, and was diagnosed with lung cancer. Money being no object, the Stewart family called in experts from many parts of the world to see if they could save their friend."

"To make a long story short," Stewart grimly announced to Merta, "the final decision was that nothing could be done for the poor fellow. The only thing they had to recommend was that he be provided with a case of whiskey to ease his pain and suffering. I remember, I remember ever so clearly, how helpless we all were, just standing there looking at our friend, now doomed to an agonizing death. Not willing to believe their verdict, I asked the experts: Is there not *someone, somewhere,* or *something* that can help him? Don't you know anyone, anywhere in the world, who could offer something better than just a case of whiskey?

"They shook their shoulders and said: 'No!'

"So I repeated: 'Anybody! I don't care if he uses a mixture of Coca Cola and pigeon droppings, I mean anyone with some ideas, as crazy as they might seem. Anyone at all!'

"But they hadn't anyone to suggest. Well, on the spot, I swore an oath that I would devote a great part of my life to seeking out, anywhere I might find anyone who could offer some chance, any chance better than what those experts had to offer! When Gaston Naessens came to my attention, I saw in him just such a person and that's why he has my backing."

As impressed with Stewart's story as he was, there was something that, as Jan Merta put it, "completely amazed me." That was Stewart's being unable to tell him exactly what Naessens was doing, exactly what his theory and his methods were all about, or whether what he was up to was of any value. "I could almost tangibly feel," Jan told me, "the foundation director's immense frustration when he said that, no matter how hard he had tried, he had been unable to find, in any academic institution, including many university hospitals, any research director or department head, even among those well known to him, who would open-mindedly take a research interest in Naessens's research or discoveries. In a kind of confessional, he said: 'Each time I bring up the name Naessens, the atmosphere becomes so frigid that it brings further conversation to a screeching halt. Even my offers of ample funding for research don't elicit the slightest reaction, not to speak of any enthusiasm.'"

One can get a good idea of Stewart's opinion of the Banerjees, and their dogma-tainted research, by his next statement to Merta: "I can say categorically that most scientific researchers with whom I have had to deal are highly opinionated, arrogant, and condescending, and have built-in, insurmountable prejudices. While showing not the slightest desire to learn

Naessens's techniques, they were nevertheless not loath to brush aside his findings without having any knowledge whatsoever about them." At that point in their conversation, Stewart paused and, looking directly into Merta's eyes, asked if he might be able to help him.

"How?" asked Jan.

"Listen," Stewart replied, "I know a great deal about your past activities. It is clear to me that you are a fighter, that you have an open mind and, more importantly, no vested interest in the outcome of Naessens's work, because your field of interest is entirely different. On the other hand, with your academic training and varied experiences, your laboratory skills, and your scientific integrity, I believe you are in a good position to assess for me what Naessens is doing, whether it is right, or wrong, and whether he has developed something important or not. So, if you can become involved, I would greatly appreciate it."

David Stewart was not exaggerating about Merta's technical expertise, and particularly about his bacteriological and microbiological training. The foundation director knew that Jan had, for instance, as far back as 1970–1971, made painstaking analyses of thousands upon thousands of blood samples, taken from both animal and human, to assess such hormone levels within them as those of cortisone, corticosterone, and androgens. As one who had learned "competitive protein binding" techniques newly developed at a local Montréal hospital, he was at that time one of a small handful of individuals around the world first to use such methods.

The foundation director also knew that Jan had taken highly intensive instruction in the Department of Bacteriology at Aberdeen's Forest Hill Hospital, particularly as it related to microbiological problems associated with long-term "saturation diving." As Merta told me, "This very practical training led to important 'field applications,' meaning I had to take swabs from divers' ears, culture them in proper media, and analyze them under the microscope to see with what kind of gram-negative bacteria I was having to deal. I had to distinguish these from natural ear flora, then use sensitivity tests to determine which antibiotics were required to effect treatment. All in all, a complex and highly precise technique."

Stewart further learned that, working on his own initiative, Merta had researched the life and work of Frederick Koch, M.D., an American physician who had developed, prior to World War II, a cancer-curing product called glyoxylide. The campaign mounted by the American Medical Association to destroy Koch's work was termed by the nationally prominent syndicated columnist Drew Pearson "the worst scandal in American medical history." Finally, in the 1940s, the scandal sent Koch to exile in Brazil for the rest of his life. After more than two years of assiduous searching, Merta had located, in Florida, one of the few people who had worked with Koch and who knew how to prepare his medicinal, learned the technique, and successfully prepared it on his own.

"I was complimented by Stewart's request," Merta told me in his Ottawa home, spangled with sealed and beribboned certificates attesting to a noble lineage that would allow him, if he so chose, to bear the titles of count, duke, and prince. "I felt I was being offered a splendid opportunity to learn more about Naessens's work. So I accepted Stewart's request but threw in: 'I don't think Naessens has told anyone exactly how he has gone about his work. So I strongly doubt he'll be willing to tell me!'"

"Don't worry," Stewart reassured Merta, "I'll arrange it."

"And, to my frank amazement, he did," continued Merta to me, "so I decided to devote the whole of my three-week annual leave from my Scottish job to work with Naessens in his lab. In the autumn of 1978, I moved temporarily to Rock Forest, staying in an upstairs room in their house, and immediately took up the task. Naessens revealed everything to me. He taught me how to use his microscope, how it was built and worked, and how to analyze what I saw in it, to the point where, quite independently of him, I could read any kind of blood samples, both human and animal, and determine the stages to which the somatid cycle had developed.

"He showed me how to extract somatids from fresh blood, how to culture them in vitro, and how to reinject them back into the blood of animals. Together, we did many experiments, all of which I vividly remember, one of them with Kelectomine, the same one you told me Dr. Lipinski did in Boston, and the ones with rabbits to show that, following body-to-body somatid transfer, the animals' hair would change color and they could mutually accept skin grafts with no sign of rejection.

"After many days of work, we finally focused on his main product, 714-X, last in a line of pharmaceuticals he had invented, and the most effective to date. He taught me how to prepare it. Working under his coaching and supervision, I then prepared about a gallon of his camphorminium chloride solution, which was relatively easy to do.

"I was grateful to Naessens for allowing me to have this experience. When I left his laboratory, I was confident that I understood the whole of his philosophy and theory, as well as all the practical aspects of his work.

"When I returned to Scotland, I had access to a microbiological lab and all its equipment. So, in time, I began to recreate all of the products that Naessens had taught me how to make. Once one has mastered the techniques, they are all fairly easy to reproduce.

"Then, all on my own, I once again reproduced the 714-X. In 1980, I came across a male dog, an old Labrador retriever, in the last stages of cancer that had afflicted its mammary glands, a dog whose veterinarian said was completely beyond help and had only a few weeks to live. When I first saw the dog, he was lying on a sofa, unable to move, with listless eyes, a high temperature, and dry skin. From his underbelly hung a huge pendulous tumor, the size of a small melon, and weighing nearly three pounds. The dog's owner, the proprietor of a large Scots manor house converted into a hotel, was so fond of the animal that he refused to put him to sleep because he wanted him to be able to pass his last days in the home he loved.

"When I told the owner I had a product that might help his dog, he told me to try anything I wanted. So I gave the dog twenty-one injections of the 714-X I had made, one each day as specified by Naessens, injecting the product into the dog's lymph system, via one of its nodes, as also specified. To his owner's, and his veterinarian's, utter astonishment, the dog completely recovered. I have photos to prove this. The tumor, no longer cancerous, and reduced to a benign sac of 'mush,' was surgically excised. In his gratitude, the dog owner gave me a case of expensive Moët et Chandon champagne as a Christmas present, a remarkably generous gift for any Scotsman."

When Dr. Jan Merta de Velehrad came to Montréal to report on his preparation of 714-X and his treatment of the dog, his documentation, including the "before and after treatment" photos of the dog itself, convinced Stewart that Jan's carefully performed work had provided concrete evidence that Naessens's 714-X might really work, however "anecdotal" the results might appear to some.

Here we should pause to say that the word *anecdotal* is loaded, in present-day scientific circles, with a meaning that has little to do with its true etymological root. In classical Greek, *anekdotos* simply means "unpublished." This would imply that when Merta reported the facts to Stewart, they were no longer "anecdotal." But, for one reason or another, the term has come to mean "unsubstantiated," or "devoid of sufficient evidence to constitute proof." So it has joined with the word "artifact" to dispose of new scientific advances. One could just as well say that record-setting victories in the Olympic Games are "anecdotal" because sufficient studies have never been made on the accuracy of the timepieces used to clock them. It could remind us, also, of the endless protests by the American government and others that the effects of acid rain on the environment are "anecdotal" because "scientific" proofs of them have not been "one hundred percent" established.

"The next time I was in Montréal," Jan told me in 1989, "I had dinner with David Stewart and his wife at their home. During our conversation, I came to realize how much Stewart's support of Naessens was, above all, based on the idea that 'a last chance' was indeed worth backing, as well as on a driving curiosity on the part of a man wealthy enough to afford, and indulge in, one.

"I have abiding admiration for David Stewart that, in spite of the years of hostility he encountered on the part of dozens of 'experts,' he never wavered in his support of Gaston Naessens and his research. This, I am convinced, is because Stewart doubted the medical establishment, the cancer 'dictatorship,' could, or would, ever produce a positive result, despite the millions and millions of dollars he, and many others, had poured into trying to find a solution."

It is Dr. Merta's firm opinion that his experience with Naessens's work and its underlying philosophy, and his treatment of the Labrador dog, went far to provide David Stewart with the additional energy and courage needed to continue backing Gaston Naessens and to fund a second round of academic experiments with dogs—and cows—in the years 1982–1985. But before taking up that costly second effort, at Guelph University, in Guelph, Ontario, we must turn our attention to another project, which, though lesser in scope, is most remarkable just because the Naessenses were not made aware of its existence until it was brought out at Naessens's trial.

Chapter 9
Guelph

The highly toxic chemotherapy, often defended by orthodox medicine with such biting aggressiveness, is in fact no more suited as a cancer therapy than a zeppelin would be to cope with a massive trans-Atlantic airlift. Only a few may reach the other shore, and at enormous cost.

Hans A. Nieper, M.D.,
Revolution in Technology, Medicine, and Society

All the foregoing has given readers some idea of what Naessens was up against throughout the 1970s: If carried out with skill and goodwill, most aspects of his pioneering work were easily replicable. But, when beset by dogmatic attitudes, their very basis was undermined a priori, whether through error or intent.

We now return momentarily to the courtroom, where, after the second weekend break, Ducharme continued his rundown of MacDonald-Stewart Foundation projects funded with the aim of proving out that work. Two of these are ordered in the sequence of their pursuit, rather than in that of their presentation in court, which failed to follow a historical order because of difficulties in scheduling the appearance of witnesses. By presenting the two projects and questioning the individual researchers in charge of them, the prosecution's chief aim, as it had been in the case of Dent's testimony, was to expose the utter worthlessness of all of Naessens's claims.

The first project had its inception on 12 August 1980, when Naessens was visited in Rock Forest by David Stewart, who still hoped that some qualified member of the medical corps and the cancer establishment might as expertly master

Naessens's lab techniques, and as fruitfully apply them to a cancerous animal, as had Jan Merta de Velehrad.

The man recommended to him by the Hôtel Dieu Hospital's Dr. Yvan Boivin was one of the same hospital's staffers, Gaétan Jasmin, a doctor and professor of medicine whom Stewart brought along with him to Rock Forest. At dinner in the Provençal, a French restaurant cozily lit by a fireplace in a typical French-Canadian stone house on the edge of town, Jasmin, at Stewart's behest, began discussing with Naessens the possibility of setting up a protocol for *preliminary* experiments with cancer-infected rats. As agreed upon, their limited aim was to determine which dose levels of 714-X, and which injection routes into the little animals' bodies, might best cure them of artificially induced lymphomas.

Pinpointing the main difficulty connected with Jasmin's proposal, Naessens asked the doctor whether he thought it would be possible to develop a special technique to allow the rats to be intralymphatically injected, since that was the only method that could assure the experiments' success. Jasmin replied that, though the problem was a difficult one, due to the extremely small size of the creatures' lymph nodes, he was confident that it could be solved. Over dessert, he promised that, when he had found the solution, he would mail Naessens a protocol, including all details about the technique, so that the biologist himself could repeat experiments along the same lines as those pursued in Montréal.

No such protocol was ever sent to Rock Forest. Since Naessens received no further communication from Jasmin, he naturally concluded that the project they had discussed together had been abandoned due to the fact that the doctor had discovered that intralymphatic injection of rats had proved impossible.

Imagine his surprise, therefore, when, during his court testimony, Ducharme handed to the prosecutor a ninety-seven-page booklet, *1er Colloque Médical David MacDonald-*

Stewart 1982. The booklet contained eight articles devoted to orthodox cancer research, plus one more, authored by Gaétan Jasmin, "Action of the Compound 714-X on the Growth of Lymphosarcoma in the Rat." It was the first time in his life that Gaston Naessens had ever learned of its publication. The short article made plain that Jasmin, though he knew full well that intralymphatic injection was indispensable to obtain any positive results, had unilaterally decided, without ever informing Naessens, to inject the rats, either subcutaneously or into what is called a peritoneum, a sac that surrounds all the organs in an animal's abdomen. Jasmin evidently reasoned, or hoped, that, because this sac contains lymphatic ganglia, some of them might somehow absorb some of the product.

It was clear that, just as had the Banerjees at McMaster University, Jasmin at the Hôtel Dieu believed that, once mandated by Stewart, he could proceed not as Naessens, but as he himself, "saw fit."

As misconstrued as it was, Jasmin's whole year-long experimentation was doomed to failure in advance. And fail it did. Though, as had been agreed with Naessens, it was conceived only as a "preliminary trial," it was not followed up. Instead, its results were rushed into print and published in Stewart's 1982 *Colloquium* booklet with the conclusion: "Our results indicate that the antitumoral agent exercised no significant effect." Once again, the word "antitumoral" indicates that Jasmin, like all his fellow cancer researchers, could not free himself of the persuasion that, to be effective, any cancer-combative product had to have a cytotoxic—or, to use another word erroneously characterizing it in Jasmin's opening paragraph, a "chemotherapeutic"—action. His conclusions showed that, whether he wanted to or not, the cancer "expert" had not the faintest idea of the real purpose of 714-X.

This did not prevent Jasmin from taking the stand to summarize orally the negative conclusions written into his article. Nor did it prevent the prosecutor from holding his "expert" witness's testimony up to the jury as a convincing proof of Naessens's ineptitude and ignorance.

Jasmin declared that his rats had been injected intraperitoneally, rather than intralymphatically, simply because "we decided it was not necessary." Cross-questioned by Chapdelaine as to whether he had ever consulted, or worked, with Naessens during the course of his experimentation, the doctor only blithely noted that there "had been no reason to do so." Though the whole above-described background to Jasmin's project was left out of his testimony, and therefore never brought out in court, had the jurors known of it they would certainly have discounted Jasmin's conclusions almost, if not completely, in toto.

Completely oblivious to the gross error involved, Québec newspapers, the following morning, all ran versions of a headline printed in the Sherbrooke English-language daily *The Record:* "714-X Didn't Help Rats Either." The *Record's* reporter, Ann McLaughlin, picking up Jasmin's comment that the product had *no effect on cancer cells,* even went as far as to wrongly attribute the words in her headline to Gaston Naessens himself.

The word "either" in the headline referred to the second project, also begun in 1980, about which testimony had already been offered in court, to the effect that 714-X had failed with dogs. Partly conceived in David Stewart's mind as a result of Dr. Merta's successful treatment of the Labrador retriever in Scotland, it was run, until 1984, at Guelph University's School of Veterinary Medicine in Guelph, Ontario. It actually began not with dogs, but with a cow. The animal in question, a prize-winning member of a rare European breed, had hardly become pregnant than she fell ill with what was diagnosed as a bovine cancer so serious that she was predicted to die before she could settle her calf. Because he wanted to do anything at all to save the valuable animal, Dr. Victor E.

"Ted" Valli, D.V.M., professor of pathology and senior member of the school's faculty, accepted Stewart's proposal that the first thing to do was to try to save the cow, and her fetus, with 714-X.

The cow survived to produce a beautiful and healthy little offspring and went back to her barn, and her pastures. Valli's letter to David Stewart, dated 16 July 1980, read, in part: "We have a cow with lymphoma on treatment who should have been in the terminal stages of the disease and who has returned to a normal attitude and food intake." He also mentioned that a "very skilled mycoplasmologist at our institution has been able consistently to isolate an unknown organism from tumor-bearing cases. . . . She believes this organism to be a mycoplasma of an unknown type." So at least one specialist seemed to have come across one of the fungoid forms in Naessens's somatid cycle. But there is no evidence in the record that further efforts were made to find out what this "unknown" organism could possibly represent.

If things had so auspicious a start at Guelph, one of the reasons appeared to be that, when he first came to the veterinary school, 714-X's inventor was introduced, not under his own real name, but under a pseudonym, Lamontagne. Stewart had decided on the alias because he wanted, at all costs, to avoid the "knee-jerk" situation, as described to Jan Merta, in which academically trained people working in the area of cancer research automatically evinced open hostility whenever the name "Naessens" was mentioned.

But, just as at McMaster University, a Stewart-funded project that had been so promisingly launched began to founder when, in the course of its pursuit, main responsibility for it was turned over to a second researcher. And, just before the experimental riders changed horses in midstream, the "cat" of Naessens's true name somehow escaped from its "bag," and became known to the veterinary school's staff. From then onward, things at Guelph ran nowhere but "downhill."

It was not Dr. Valli but the second researcher who was put on the stand by prosecutor Melançon. Dr. Ronald Carter, since become a well-funded researcher on human cancer, had, at the time the Stewart-commissioned studies were being performed in Guelph, been a veterinary school student.

Instead of attempting to summarize and comment upon Carter's interminable testimony, which, like that of others before him, took the flight of a headless chicken rather than a crow, we shall refer to what was reported about it in French in the Sherbrooke *Tribune*, and in English in the Sherbrooke *Record*. "A clinical study," reads the article,

suggested that the experimental product 714-X had no effect in the treatment of lymphatic tumors in dogs. This conclusion was founded on an evaluation of eight dogs which received this treatment within the framework of study done at Guelph. No dog had the benefit of remission, and all of them died of cancer.

That is what was reported yesterday by Dr. Ronald Carter, who participated in the study in which three dogs received injections of the experimental product *intravenously*, then, following new directives, the others were similarly treated *intralymphatically*.

So, just as Jasmin had decided to ignore the injection route so necessary to success, Carter, for whatever reasons, also began his experiments while totally ignoring the crucial injection mode.*

---

*In a deposition of 5 February 1985, prepared for investigator Luc Grégoire, *Bureau des enquêtes criminelles*, in Sherbrooke, Valli wrote: "I indicated to [Carter's] Supervisory Committee that I had talked to Mr. Lamontagne by telephone and that we had been instructed to try twenty-one consecutive daily injections into *affected lymph nodes* [emphasis supplied]." The text of the deposition continues: "This conversation was carried out in French through an

Though new directives were given by Naessens himself to change the injection route to the correct intralymphatic one, for lack of other precise instructions, the dosage, as reported by the *Tribune,* "varied from 0.5 milliliters per kilogram of body weight for the first intravenous method to 0.02 for the second intralymphatic one." Nor was that the only inexplicable variable. Though only a limited number of sick dogs were experimented on, they variously received, apparently haphazardly, anywhere between three and twenty-six injections.

How anyone could make much of the newspaper account as far as comprehending what was going on in the "topsy-turvy" Guelph experimentation, was a question never raised in its text. In terms of the dogs' survival time, it concluded, Carter had stated that 714-X was a far less successful treatment than chemotherapy. Even worse, he added, Naessens's product had caused anorexia (lack of appetite, and lassitude) and depression in the animals, as well as pain in their lymph nodes. More caustically, the Sherbrooke *Record* featured Carter's statement that the dogs had done so poorly with the 714-X injections that his veterinary teaching hospital colleagues had gone to the lengths of hiding prospective subjects from him. This was why it had taken over three years to run tests on only eight dogs for a two- to three-week period. As for the *Journal de Montréal,* its headline on its report on Carter's testimony said it all: "The Ineffectiveness of 714-X Has Been Proved!" Anyone who read the dire conclusion might well have predicted, at least at that point, that Gaston Naessens was headed into a jail cell.

---

interpreter. As a result of problems with the language, the initial animals in the study were *given an overdose* . . . [emphasis also supplied]." This footnote has been inserted here to indicate not only how communications on proper experimentation were sorely lacking, but that they were further complicated and distorted by Naessens's lack of command of the English language.

Not reported to the public, because, as previously noted, their publication is legally disallowed, were more *Voir Dire* portions of the testimony during which defense attorney Chapdelaine made Carter confess that, in fact, he had never discussed any of his work with his client, the foundation, but had "followed verbal directives from his immediate supervisor, Valli." This could not be confirmed, however, because, inexplicably, Valli himself declined to appear in court to back up Carter's claim. Whether or not Valli would have undermined Carter's allegation, the issue of his nonappearance was left shrouded in no little mystery. Could it have been that, had he been called to testify, this senior veterinary scientist would have felt himself to be in a difficult position and constrained to raise specters laid to rest more than a half a decade earlier?

Most disturbing of all, with regard to the Guelph goings-on, was Carter's allegation that the cow that, together with her calf, had been saved by 714-X, had been *misdiagnosed*—that is, she never had the cancer she was supposed to have had in the first place. It seemed that, in hindsight, any success obtained with 714-X could be written off to prior diagnostic error.

The tortuous aspects of all this testimony were finally sorted out by Judge Péloquin when he ruled that Carter could tell what he had told under *Voir Dire* all over again to the jury, but with exceptions.

"Voici!" he began with an introductory word that is the French equivalent of "Here it is!" "It is certain that Carter's experimentation was done according to instructions, and the court realizes that they ran into difficulties. In its ensemble, Carter's expertise has a certain probing value because it was done with the intent of discovering whether or not 714-X had a beneficial effect on dogs. But this probing value vis-à-vis *humans* will be up to the jury. So I believe this proof must be admitted only with restriction."

This meant that Carter could not refer to his superior, Dr. Valli, in any support of his own testimony because it would be "hearsay." "If the Crown wants to hear from Valli, then it must call him," ruled the judge.

And, though Chapdelaine held that Valli *should* testify, the prosecutor, insisting that he had no intention of calling the veterinarian, added snidely: "Who can oblige me to have him here, certainly not my confrere!"

The judge retorted: "I'll be forced to tell the jury that!" To which Melançon curtly replied: "I'll take that risk!"

During his cross-examination, Chapdelaine embarrassed Carter not a little by asking a number of precise questions about the timing of this or that phase of the experimentation on these or those animals. To all of which, the witness, his hands now nervously twitching, a bit weakly replied that he was unable to remember the "exact chronology" of events.

Carter brushed aside Chapdelaine's next question on whether his report had been published in a scientific journal with the disdainful statement that, because there was already so much positive material being published on cancer, "negative results," such as those he had obtained, should not "burden the literature."

What was next, almost incredibly, revealed was that, though no report had been published in a scientific journal, a long negative ninety-nine-page summary of Carter's negative findings, also completely unknown to Naessens, had been prepared for the MacDonald-Stewart Foundation, or at least ostensibly so. The fact that the report did not bear a date in 1984, the year the Guelph project had ended, but September 1985, was astounding. The sloppily printed pages of the summary indicate that it was gotten up in great haste only after the police investigation of Naessens. Could this have been because the report was made more for the police investigation than for any other reason? At any rate, it ended up by "burdening" not any scientific or medical archive, but a legal one.

It was on Wednesday, 22 November, that the next prosecution witness took the stand. He was none other than the cancer specialist Yvan Boivin, M.D., through whose office, at the Hôtel Dieu Hospital, the MacDonald-Stewart monies, destined for Naessens himself, had all along been channeled, as they continue to be to this day.

Philosophically speaking, two remarks made by Boivin during his testimony seemed singularly, and shockingly, impressive. The first was "I am orthodox in my view and *therefore biased!*" The second, with reference to Naessens's microscope, was "When I first looked into it about ten years ago, *I saw a whole new world!* So new, I really didn't know what I was beholding!"

What is strange, beyond all imagination, is that, having seen that "new world," Boivin never bothered to take a second look. Though he also stated, almost parenthetically, that his own cytological interest led him to believe that the microscope might be able to solve a thorny problem, that of accurately assessing cells that are becoming, but have not yet become, cancerous, he never took the initiative of commissioning Naessens to attack that problem. He therefore might be compared to one of the church cardinals who, after looking once through Galileo's telescope, did not deign to look twice, so shocking were its revelations to his limited view of the world around him.

What can explain this kind of disinterest on the part of a self-proclaimed "scientist"? While discussing the testimony of Dr. Lorenzo Haché, with its references to "marginal" research, we brought up Dr. Beverly Rubik's article dealing with the enigmas and difficulties facing "frontier" scientists such as Naessens. In order to try to shed some light on Boivin's apathy with respect not only to a "second look," but to any in-depth investigation of new knowledge, let us again quote Rubik's incisive article:

The saga of the recent work in France by Jacques Benveniste in immunology [exactly the field of Naessens's preoccupations] provides a living example of such difficulties. Dr. Benveniste is a prominent scientist and director of immunology at a national institute of medical research near Paris. He has published several dozen research papers, some of which are citation classics. In June 1988, he published a paper together with several others in a prestigious scientific journal demonstrating the effect on cells of antibody solutions so dilute that they no longer contained any measurable amount of substance. This suggests that water has "memory."

Since this paper shook the foundations of the established sciences of chemistry, pharmacology and medicine, the publishers had serious editorial reservations. In an unprecedented action the journal editor sent an investigating team consisting of himself, an expert in scientific fraud, and a magician famous for debunking parapsychological research, to the French laboratory. After only three days work, they concluded that the effect did not exist. An expert immunologist was not even present! This was such a crude attempt to disprove Benveniste's claims that the journal was forced to let him protest his report.

Given Rubik's account, could anyone wonder that Naessens, out on the "frontier" since his twenties, opted to push forward with his research while *never* opting to get it published anywhere, knowing in advance that his discoveries would be accorded exactly the same inquisitorial treatment as Benveniste's?

In her article, Rubik sadly shows that, despite increasing evidence to support the Benveniste effect, a magician — the "Amazing Randi" who took part in debunking it — was given the annual award of the prestigious American Physics Society (APS) for this effort in 1989. Given the optical anomalies associated with Naessens's microscope, how would these be greeted today by APS members as a group? And if they sent a "magician" to debunk it, would he be given another prize? Can any of this possibly explain why Naessens has been content to keep his microscope "quiet" for over forty years, and just use it to get on with his other discoveries?

Let us read another passage from Rubik's article:

> The Jacques Benveniste *affaire* illustrates dramati-
> cally the reception that new ideas and findings some-
> times receive in science today. Despite the fact that
> "science" exists to reveal new data, discoveries consid-
> ered anomalous or incomprehensible [like Boivin's "whole
> new world"] by current scientific understanding are not
> warmly received by the contemporary scientific estab-
> lishment. In fact, throughout the history of science, truly
> novel discoveries and ideas contradicting those of the es-
> tablishment [such as those of Gaston Naessens] were
> often dismissed, or ignored.
>
> Kepler was accused of introducing occultism when
> he proposed that the moon controls the motion of the
> tides. Lord Kelvin held that X rays were a hoax. Barbara
> McClintock toiled in isolation most of her long life with
> little support, unraveling the mysteries of the transposi-
> tion of genes, until recently when she was finally awarded
> the Nobel Prize.

All this is set down to give readers some additional understanding of what a research giant like Naessens really
faces, in the light of past or contemporary history, from men
of different stature, such as the Dents, Jasmins, Carters,
Boivins, and Roys of this world.

Toward the end of his testimony, Boivin revealed that
when, despite all the setbacks, David Stewart insisted that research on Naessens's science continue, and that he, Boivin, had

strongly recommended against it, Stewart had chided him with being "stubbornly orthodox." This declaration evoked from prosecutor Melançon a vulgar guffaw: "Orthodox, fancy that!"

As if picking up Melançon's cue, Boivin went on: "I told Stewart, then and there, that there were sixteen thousand physicians in Québec, and forty-five thousand in Canada, all of whom could be considered *orthodox.*" Just as if Stewart were not already aware of that fact, and as if their very numbers were the final argument as to what might be worthwhile in the pursuance of frontier medical research!

The prosecutor had now "shot his bolt." Whether, in the jurors' ears, he had hit his target and wounded his intended victim gravely or mortally only they would ultimately judge. Certainly, they would remember Ducharme's reply when he was asked by Melançon why research into 714-X had finally come to an end in 1985: "I imagine it was because nothing of value ever came out of it. While he was alive, Stewart pursued it down first one avenue, then another, 'blind alleys' all, or so it would seem. He always wanted to 'keep the door ajar,' make one more *démarche.* But, as you can see, from the 1985 Guelph report, the product was ineffective. . . . "

And they would remember Melançon's tone of triumph when he cut in to trumpet: "*Ineffective!* 714-X . . . Camphorminium chloride . . . was *ineffective!*" One could have believed that, right there, he had won his battle.

Now that his performance was over, it was time for Melançon to cede his place on the legal stage to Chapdelaine. Thousands of cancer victims all over the world, had they known about the trial in Sherbrooke, surely would have awaited the defense attorney's retort with more than a little anticipation.

Chapter 10
The Defense

*It was not, and would not be, leaks that would do us
in, but suppression of the facts of what was happening in
the world. Nothing is more difficult to report than the
truth, and few, indeed, are those who want to read
the tough, harsh words of reality.*
Harrison Salisbury, in his autobiography
A Journey for Our Times

It was late in the afternoon when Chapdelaine opened his
case for the defense and things began to liven up following
the long hours of tedious, and often boring, testimony by
prosecution witnesses.

We have seen that the defense attorney's strategy was
not to confront his adversary on the narrow issue of the chief
count against his client, that of contributing to the death of
a patient. As his witnesses trooped, one by one, to the stand,
it became clearer and clearer that his real aim was to set the
whole of Naessens's lifelong research in the broadest possible
perspective and to show that his product, 714-X, if administered by knowing minds and capable hands, had produced
startlingly successful results with cancer victims, not just
rats, dogs, or cows, but living, breathing, suffering human
beings.

Chapdelaine began by stating to the jurors, who now
appeared less lethargic and more "electrically" awake than
before, that though Gaston Naessens had the right, as does
any defendant, *not* to testify, he in fact *would* testify. "Why?"
asked Chapdelaine rhetorically. And, to answer the question,
he declared that what was being brought out during the present trial was a problem, enormous in its importance for so-

ciety, whose members are everywhere dying of cancer with
each passing day.

To counter the weight of the prosecution's medical "experts," whose often abysmal ignorance of Naessens's whole
new science he had been able subtly to reveal, Chapdelaine
called a thirty-five-year-old French doctor of medicine, Michel
Fabre, who had flown the Atlantic to offer his testimony.

To cut straight into the heart of the matter, the difference between the approach of thousands of orthodox cancerologists—or *oncologists,* as they are more technically known—
to healing, and the almost diametrically opposed approach
of one individual, Gaston Naessens, Fabre began with an analogy, as simple as it was apt. Likening the appearance of cancer
cells in the body to the appearance of a swarm of mosquitoes in an outdoor locale, the doctor said that traditional medicine sought only to destroy offending cells—through surgery,
radiation, or chemotherapy—just as one might attempt to get
rid of the mosquito swarm by spraying it with insecticides.*
This was a hopeless task, Fabre continued, because, just as
mosquitoes come out of a *swamp* favorable to their breed-
ing and generation, so cancerous cells develop in a bodily
milieu, or *terrain,* favoring such development. It was therefore Naessens's aim, not to seek to annihilate the mosquitoes (the cancer cells) one by one, but to eradicate the swampy
conditions that had led them to engender in the first place.
Chronic disease was closely linked to a morasslike condition
in the body.

---

*To return to Louis Pasteur, whose "germ theory" of disease gained
ascendancy for nearly a century: Pasteur was reported to have said,
on his deathbed, with reference to the ideas of the eminent French
physiologist Claude Bernard, who championed the notion that the
terrain was more significant than germs in the onset of disease: "Bernard a raison . . . le terrain is tout! Le microbe n'est rien!" (Bernard
is right . . . the terrain is everything! The microbe is nothing!). This
confession, unfortunately, was not heard beyond the bedroom walls.

As for Naessens's principal discovery of the somatid and the cycle of microbes into which it developed, all made possible by the invention of a unique microscope, the physician stated that he believed that this discovery was more important than any made by Pasteur in the past century. What Naessens had unearthed, he asserted, was no less than the material foundation, the physical basis, for life itself, and, more esoterically or metaphysically, for what is known as the "etheric" body, without which the physical body, which it interpenetrates, would be only inert matter, as it indeed becomes at death, when the soul takes leave of it.

At this point, as well they might, the expressions on the jurors' faces ranged from highly intent to rapt. And it came to me that one would have to travel far indeed, perhaps to the world's end, to hear similar words issue from the mouth of a medical professional in a court of law. I will go farther, to say that I believe this ringing testimony from a doctor, under oath to tell "the truth, the whole truth, and nothing but the truth," may, when, and if, it becomes widely known, represent a blueprint for a new medical philosophy concerning the true nature of humanity. As a professional physician, Michel Fabre had, without doubt, made a statement of the greatest historical importance, one that can never be expunged by materialists or mechanists from the record.

Chapdelaine must also have been impressed, but, as a legal expert dealing with facts, rather than opinion, he was evidently also a trifle alarmed at the philosophical heights to which his witness was soaring. Shortly after the court session came to an end, I heard him gently cautioning Fabre not to go "too far" or be "too eloquent" in his support of Naessens's research. "Don't overdo it," he admonished. "That might only hurt our case. Stick to the subject at hand."

The warning notwithstanding, it may have been fortuitous that the jurors, retired to their homes to rest from their labors, had been left with a series of powerful reflections delivered in so simple a language that no special erudition was required for their understanding. In a just few minutes of testimony, Fabre seemed to have elevated the whole theme, or nexus, of the trial to a higher plane and carried those jurors, or at least some of them, up to that same level.

When the trial resumed early Monday morning, Dr. Fabre, looking just as "elfin" as he had the previous Friday, was led by Maître Chapdelaine over the history, the "trail," of how he had first been introduced to Gaston Naessens and his research. The contact had been made through Sam Cohen, a Parisian businessman, whose wife, Claire Nuer, when only in her forties, had been afflicted with a melanoma of the eye, a particularly lethal cancer that usually rapidly spreads to the brain and other bodily organs. After doctors, whom, in her desperation, she had consulted, one after another, in Paris, London, and San Francisco, all recommended that she have the eye removed from its socket, she refused. Through Simone Brousse, who for years had written a column on "alternative" medicine for the French edition of the internationally known *Vogue* magazine, Claire was directed to Gaston Naessens and, within a year, saw her cancer condition disappear.

After meeting Claire Nuer, Fabre, as the son and grandson of eminently respected physicians, was as cautious as the medically orthodox traditions of his family had taught him to be. Returning home to the Massif Central, a mountainous region in the heart of France, he consulted with his father, who, hardly able to believe his son's report about recovery from melanoma, decided to take the train for Paris and "see for himself." Impressed by what he had seen, the elder doctor saw no obstacle with regard to the younger one pursuing the matter further.

With reference to Nuer's case, Fabre addressed another subtle point linked to the above-mentioned dual, and opposite, approaches to the treatment of cancer. Stating that, while medical orthodoxy holds that "cure" of cancer can be said to have taken place only after *all* traces of tumors, or cancerous cells, have disappeared from the body, he noted that Madame Nuer's ocular tumor, treated with 714-X, had actually *not* disappeared but, as proved by "scans," was seen to have atrophied, its soft tissues having hardened and become "sclerotic."

This was an important point, because, according to orthodox cancer philosophy, tumors, atrophied or not, are usually recommended for surgical excision. As it exists, the cancer establishment simply cannot believe that tumor cells, as in the case of Jan Merta de Velehrad's Labrador retriever, can be reduced to harmlessness by a bodily immune system strengthened by Naessens's method.

Chapdelaine drew Dr. Fabre out on the history of his own treatment of French patients with 714-X, patients whose medical dossiers he had brought with him in case they should be required as evidence to prove his allegations. One case he cited was that of a man who came down with lung cancer in 1988, refused to be operated, and instead took the 714-X at Dr. Fabre's recommendation and administration. "He's now in perfect shape!" Fabre reported.

Another case brought up by Fabre was particularly important because it illustrated how 714-X can be successfully used to treat intractable degenerative diseases other than cancer. It dealt with a thirty-year-old woman with an advanced case of multiple sclerosis—known colloquially as "M.S."—from which she had suffered since 1978. Since being under 714-X treatment, the woman, said Fabre, had been making remarkable progress toward health.*

---

*In the early 1980s, I myself was personally introduced to 714-X's effectiveness in reversing an advanced case of M.S. The patient in question, a close friend and a Connecticut dental surgeon in his midfifties, had been confined to a wheelchair, where he sat helplessly and incontinently, unable to feed himself or to talk. Within ten days after 714-X treatment began, the dentist was able, for the

After Chapdelaine had drawn Fabre out on the cases he had successfully treated with Naessens's product, the defense attorney posed a question particularly relevant to the trial's broader issue. Asked how his use of an "officially unauthorized" product to treat patients was received by French medical authority, the doctor unhesitatingly replied that any doctor in France could, if not *legally*, be *ethically* guided to proceed with *any* treatment he believed would help his patients, guided, as Fabre put it, by *"soul and conscience."* With those words hardly out of his mouth, he turned to look squarely at Melançon and, with a winning smile, and almost a wink, added: "This may not appeal to the legal profession, but that's the way it is!"

Like all others present, whether pro- or anti-Naessens, I was left profoundly impressed by the candidness of Fabre's declarations, which a second time had accented spiritual aspects of medical practice and ethics that could be championed by any doctor who truly believes his oath of Hippocrates to be "Hippocratic" and not hypocritical.

Looking at his confrere, Chapdelaine said, "Your witness." Prosecutor Melançon began addressing to Doctor Fabre a series of irrelevancies, details of which can be found in the extensive court transcript. It was not so much his questions and statements that were offensive, as the insulting and mocking tone with which they were delivered. There was an exaggerated crudeness in Melançon's manner that was almost past belief, one that, in the jury's eyes, could easily have hurt whatever case he was trying to build against Michel Fabre.

Dismissing most of Fabre's testimony as so much "sob-

first time in two years, to stand unsupported and take a few steps. By the end of a twenty-one-day treatment, he was able, unaided, to walk around a table, only occasionally abetting his progress by placing his forefinger on it to assure his balance. His ex-wife, who had accompanied him to Canada, where she loyally took care of him during treatment, looked upon his recovery as a "miracle."

sister tear-jerking," Melançon, with heightened disparagement, announced that his whole case would thenceforth reside on his proof that 714-X, if it had produced any positive results whatsoever, was merely a "placebo." This implied that any patient who got well had regained his health not due to the treatment itself, but only due to his or her *belief* that the product, actually no more effective than distilled water or Coca Cola, had worked to effect a cure.

Is this not an example of exactly how "peer review," brought up in Beverly Rubik's article on "Frontier Science," disposes of new knowledge? Because a product has no "peer recognition," it must necessarily be dismissed, in this case as exerting no more than a "placebo effect." Even if that were *true*, shouldn't it be admitted that, if, as in such cases as Madame Nuer's eye melanoma, it could, and did, produce a curative effect for some as yet unexplained reason, then it had extremely powerful properties?

To add insult to injury, Melançon next launched into what seemed to me a series of arguments even more irrelevant than any of the others he had put forward. As far-fetched as it might have seemed to anyone with the barest knowledge of the subject matter raised, he began to try to relate the name *somatid* to the *somatic* part of the word "psychosomatic"! What he was trying to establish would have been anyone's guess. He appeared to be asserting that the somatid, far from being anything worthwhile, or even real, was an "artifact" connected only to "belief," founded or unfounded, and to "psychological" aspects of health, which, morbidly, often lead to "hypochondria," or, more hopefully, to "faith" in "miracle" cures.

Perhaps relying on Dr. Lorenzo Haché's suggestion that he might have seen the term somatid "somewhere" in a French book, the prosecutor, continuing in a tone of snide denigration, offered that Naessens's somatid was no discovery at all, but simply a term borrowed by the biologist from the literature.

Incensed with Melançon's manner, Chapdelaine suddenly rose in protest to request of Judge Péloquin that the trial go back into *Voir Dire* session. The jury was once again dismissed, everyone in court being requested to rise, as usual, until they had made their collective departure. The defense attorney then told the judge, in no uncertain terms, that his adversary's tone, while addressing Dr. Fabre in *contre-interrogatoire*, had been inconceivably contemptuous and rude, and that he was making a virtual "circus" of the proceedings in a behavior that should halt "forthwith."

Partially agreeing, the judge, who in tribute to his even-handedness has been complimented with the nickname "Mr. Fifty-Fifty" by Sherbrooke Superior Court lawyers who have worked under his presidency, warned the prosecutor, gently rather than harshly, to "tone down." If Melançon wanted to present the jury with his "placebo" argument, he added, he was free to do so only if he also watched that his manner be "civil."

The following witness caused a stir when he entered. Tall, and a bit stooped with fatigue, his almost totally bald head was marred by a long curved scar on its right parietal section, due to an operation for a brain tumor. Massive doses of chemotherapy had subsequently caused all his hair to drop off except for a jet-black thatch that remained on the back of his skull. In Québec, the fifty-one-year-old Gérald Godin is as well known as any minister in a national government, or any ranking member of the British Parliament or the United States Congress. Having served Québec in both capacities, Godin, who shortly before his court appearance had run for office to regain his seat as Québec parliament deputy from Montréal's Mercier district, is also a well-known poet and ardent fighter for Québec's independence from the rest of Canada. When he took the stand, he was therefore familiar to everyone in the courtroom, the more so since the popular, color-illustrated weekly magazine *Sept Jours*, in its issue of 2 December 1989, had just come out on the newsstands with an article entitled: "Vaincre mon cancer: La bataille de Gérald Godin, ex-ministre" (To Conquer My Cancer: The Battle of Ex-Minister Gérald Godin). On its cover was the sadfaced Godin with the arms of his paramour, well-known Québécoise singer Pauline Julien, draped lovingly around his shoulders.

In 1984, the article reported, Godin had undergone an operation that left him partially paralyzed on the left side of his body, afflicted with epileptic fits, and, worst of all, unable to speak. "It's the most maddening experience I ever went through in my life," he was quoted as saying. "I still go through hell if I have to talk about it . . . fear, at virtually every street corner, that I might suddenly drop dead. . . . One day, if I have enough courage, I shall write about it."

As the magazine further disclosed, the poet, orator, and journalist, during months spent learning to talk, was appalled to find that the original tumor had resurged in his head. On 17 July 1989, he consequently underwent a second brain operation, followed by intensive radiation and chemotherapy from 9 August to 28 September, the results of which produced not the slightest effect, either positive or negative.

Though obviously weakened by his long ordeal, Godin, speaking clearly and with accelerated rhythm, next told the court what the magazine, at the time it was preparing its feature article, did not know and therefore did not print: At a friend's suggestion, he had decided, as a last resort, to put himself in the hands of Gaston Naessens and take the 714-X treatment.

Most impressive was his statement—given Fabre's earlier reference to *"Âme et conscience"*—that, when he decided to tell his doctor about his decision, the medico simply answered: "Why not? It's reputed to have no side effects whatsoever."

From the end of September to the twentieth of October,

Godin received a daily intralymphatic injection of 714-X in the lymph node of his groin. "I felt no pain whatsoever," he testified, "and I regained a state in which I felt much more energetic and vigorous." So vigorous, in fact, that he was able to undertake an arduous election campaign and go on to win. On 23 October, Godin's blood was examined under Naessens's microscope. Naessens was able to tell him that his blood picture had returned to normal. Furthermore, Godin also revealed that tests with a scanner at Montréal's Nôtre Dame Hospital also revealed that a cancerous mass, which surgeons had been unable to remove from the brain, had shrunken by sixty percent.

When, at the recommendation of cancer doctors, Godin again submitted to chemotherapy, he again, as he put it, "became nauseous, and lost any zest for life as well as any appetite. So I again broke off the 'chemo' for a while and, just this morning, I've decided to take some more of Naessens's shots." As other witnesses would also do, Gérald Godin testified that Naessens had at no time promised him any cure but had limited himself to saying that the treatment would most likely strengthen his immune system and, in so doing, even assist the chemotherapy. Invited by Maître Chapdelaine to cross-examine the witness, Prosecutor Melançon declined.

One can surmise that the arrival and presence in the courtroom of a well-known literary figure and ex-minister of state, who testified he had opted for Naessens's treatment *with his doctor's blessing,* must have made quite a dent in Melançon's arguments about "placebo" effects and "psychosomatic" conditions. Further, the statement by a man of recognized probity that Naessens had never *promised* him anything went far to offset allegations by her husband and daughter that Madame Langlais had been made such a promise.

It looked as if the juggernaut of Chapdelaine's defense was really rolling and the next witness did nothing to slow its momentum, quite the contrary.

In 1981, thirty-one-year-old Gary Diamond, a business-man now living in Santa Rosa, California, had been diagnosed with the very worst form of Hodgkin's disease, a cancer that attacked his lymph nodes and spread tumors in other parts of his body. After submitting to an operation, then treatment with radiation and chemotherapy, all his doctors could promise him was no more than two years of additional survival.

In a particularly lucid testimony, delivered in English and duly translated by an official court interpreter, and in a clear, firm voice as if he were reading it from a script, this son of a doctor of medicine went over all the historical details of his case. Part of the impressive documentation Diamond supplied was a copy of a "Patient Progress Record" issued on 23 August 1989 by Marek J. Bozdech, M.D., of Santa Rosa's Kaiser Permanente Hospital. After a long description of Diamond's deteriorating condition, and treatment, the report adds:

> Prior to completing his therapy . . . [i.e., chemo-], in August 1983 he visited a scientist in Canada who offered alternative treatment based on a theory of "somatids" and the theory that stimulation of the immune system could prevent or treat cancer. Accordingly, the patient received twenty-one injections directly into the inguinal lymph nodes of a nitrogen-related compound named 714-X in gradually increasing doses over twenty-one days. Following a nine-day period of treatment, he received two more cycles of twenty-one days each. He has continued these treatments. The scientist in Canada did recommend that Mr. Diamond complete his chemotherapy, which he did in August of 1983.

This citation has been included here in full because it represents one of the first, if not *the* first, official report by an American doctor on the use of 714-X in the treatment of a difficult cancer condition. In this historically important report, the fact that the doctor assigned no more weight to 714-X's role in Diamond's recovery than he did to chemotherapy—or to vitamin C, A, and E treatment also offered Diamond under the aegis of Nobel Laureate Linus Pauling—somewhat clouds the question as to exactly which treatment was effective in Diamond's cure. Though this point would be raised in the prosecutor's final plea, he would be unable to make much of it, given the recovery from cancer of several other patients, all witnesses, who had been treated by 714-X and by no other means.

One month later, Dr. Bozdech wrote a letter, addressed to medical insurance companies on Diamond's behalf, to state: "Since the patient has now been in complete remission since 1983, the likelihood of relapse is becoming increasingly small. After five years, many physicians and oncologists would agree that patients are probably cured of their Hodgkin's disease. . . . I believe Mr. Diamond should be reevaluated on the basis of his current excellent condition and freedom of disease for purposes of insurance." As a result of Bozdech's letter, Diamond was offered full coverage by four separate medical insurance companies. About this, Diamond concluded, not without humor: "I guess that if nothing else does, the issue of a medical insurance policy, at normal premium rates, has to prove my recovery!"

Asked by Chapdelaine to place his thick medical dossier "on exhibit" for the court, Diamond willingly agreed. As in the case of Godin, Claude Melançon had no questions for the witness.

The international flavor of the case for the defense was again accented with the appearance of Chapdelaine's fourth witness. Coming from the Vorarlberg province in the western "tail" of Austria, where he works as a textile engineer, Helmuth Wallaczek, also testifying in English, told how, in 1978, he had been diagnosed with a cancerous tumor in one of his kidneys and, after heavy doses of radiation, was nevertheless found to have metastases to his liver. Several Austrian doctors had sadly informed him that his prognosis was the worst imaginable.

Through his brother, who lives in the Austrian Alpine ski-resort town of Kitzbühl and travels the world giving seminars on "New Age" topics, Helmuth learned about Gaston Naessens in faraway Québec, and flew over for treatment. Unlike Gary Diamond, he had submitted to no other form of medical intervention. The result? Ever since, he has enjoyed perfect health. Wallaczek produced a thick report from his family doctor to prove that, after repeated and seemingly endless tests of all kinds made by Austrian cancer experts in his home province, he had been declared free of cancer.

He also somewhat wryly added that his doctor, "like *all* Austrian doctors," was unable to admit that anything of which he himself was *not aware* could have any curative effect upon the disease. So he could only ascribe Walleczek's cure to "some form" of mysterious *homeopathic* treatment obtained abroad. After Wallaczek's medical file was added to the now growing stack, Melançon once again declined any cross-examination.

Chapdelaine's defense "strategy" was emerging from its depths. While he could have kept the trial going for many more days by calling dozens, or even hundreds, of patients and other witnesses, such as Dr. Boguslaw Lipinski or Dr. Jan Merta de Velehrad, he had concluded that it was not the weight of witness *numbers* that would count so much as their careful selection, geographically and professionally speaking.

So far, he had lined up a doctor of medicine from France, who had boldly committed himself to treating patients with 714-X; a widely known Québec political and literary boffin; a businessman from the western United States; and an engineer from central Europe. Three of these witnesses had indubiously affirmed that they owed lives—two of them, their *own* lives—to Gaston Naessens's treatment, and the fourth had stated that he was sure that such treatment, in the face of the failure of conventional approaches, was the only one that offered him any hope of salvation.

Having exposed the jurors to the *grand monde*, it was time to "change pace," to bring matters "closer to home," so that they might feel Naessens's successful attack on one of the world's most ravaging diseases applied not only to the "educated," or those who could afford to travel from thousands of miles away, but to anyone, perhaps themselves, if they ever came down with the dreaded affliction.

Accordingly, the next witness was an "Eastern Townships" local, Jacques Viens, a mechanic hailing from Valcourt, a town about fifteen kilometers west of Sherbrooke, small, but well known because the Québec inventor of the snowmobile, Armand Bombardier, had built a large factory in his birthplace to manufacture the vehicle.

As Jacques Lemoine's summary of Viens's testimony ran in the Sherbrooke *Tribune:*

Viens, aged only thirty-nine, told how, on 6 June last, he had had seven-eighths of his stomach surgically removed because it had become infected with cancer, which had also affected his lymph nodes.

Six days later he decided to go home to die.

Since his doctor could no longer do anything for him, and he didn't want to die so prematurely, on June 20th, he began the 714-X treatment.

Monsieur Viens said he had taken that treatment from a person within the medical corps whose name he preferred not to disclose.

In the late autumn, he went hunting for deer and moose and, five weeks ago, returned to work.

A man who, less than half a year before, had virtually been condemned to death.

From my notes:

Throughout today's testimony, it was obvious that the jurors were on the edge of their seats, riveted by what the witnesses had to say, hanging on every word. Quite the opposite from the bored looks they wore last week while forced to hear the almost endless *verbillage* of cancer experts. What did all that *verbillage* mean when here were patients, or doctors, from three foreign countries, and two from their own native Québec, one from higher "strata," one from lower, offering solid testimony that *someone, somewhere,* had come up with *something* that had put an end to cancerous pain and suffering? It is indeed a pity that David Stewart died before the trial, for he, above all, would have reveled at the notion that the "maverick" he had backed for so long was at last so triumphantly being vindicated in public.

Also, I noticed that Luc Grégoire, the "cop" who had led the whole investigation against Naessens, and who was the first significant witness at this trial, had, if not tears, at least signs of them, in his eyes while listening to parts of the patients' testimonies.

It was over the weekend of the 26–27 November that Françoise Naessens began to have personal misgivings, in fact severe doubts, that anything positive was to be gained by Chapdelaine's putting her husband on the stand. Though his voluntary testimony might, from one point of view, cast him as a brave man, with nothing to hide, ran her thinking, if he was not required by law to testify, then why should he? What possible good could come out of it?"

It was an important question, a grave one, that she put to her husband, to others, and finally to their lawyer, Conrad Chapdelaine. Grave, because, as she thought over matters, she came to the conclusion that, were Gaston called, then prosecutor Melançon might drag him, perhaps for hours, into minute detail about aspects of his research, and of his whole life, that would have little bearing on the excellent case the defense attorney had been putting up, simply by letting Naessens's patients tell the jury, on behalf of the biologist himself, what he had actually *done*, done for them, and for many, many others. Furthermore, it might give the prosecutor the chance, once again, to open up the whole "story" surrounding Madame Langlais's demise, to refresh, in the minds of the jury, the most serious charge against the defendant, namely, the possibility that he had been an accomplice to the murder of a helpless and unsuspecting woman.

Though I was not present to hear this issue discussed between Chapdelaine and the Naessenses, I gathered later from Françoise herself that the attorney had realized that, as it goes in French, *she had reason*, that "she was right," in almost every respect. Due to this fundamental change in strategy, Melançon was thus prevented from reassuming his "prosecutor's" role in the courtroom.

The ever-heightening intensity of emotion in the courtroom was lessened not a whit when, the following Monday morning, Chapdelaine next called to the stand another Québecer, who, if first impression of externals were an only guide, could easily have been taken for a senior diplomat or well-known film star. Marcel Caron, a fifty-one-year-old ex–sales manager for Heinz ("Fifty-seven Varieties"), was nattily dressed in a blue blazer that perfectly offset his well-chiseled features topped with a full head of salt-and-pepper hair.

In a voice ringing with confidence, Caron recounted how he had contracted intestinal problems in 1981. Polyps discovered in his intestine and surgically removed were one week later found to be cancerous. Never having been sick for one day in his life, Caron was advised to have an indeterminate portion of his intestine excised without delay. He adamantly refused for a variety of reasons, the most important being that his younger brother, struck down with exactly the same affliction in 1970, had consented to exactly the same operation recommended to Caron himself, only to survive for an additional six months and to die in great agony.

Luckily, Caron's wife had been successfully treated for breast cancer with 714-X as administered by Stephen Zalac. So, two days after the suggested operation had been scheduled to take place, Marcel was guided by her to Naessens's Rock Forest laboratory. Upon examining Caron's blood at the microscope, Naessens, who had not been told of the subject's condition, told him that he had a "deteriorated blood picture" (he did not mention the word "cancer") that suggested a serious weakening of his immune defense system, which could be reinforced by 714-X.

At Maître Chapdelaine's request, Caron was also led to stress that Naessens had never once promised him any cure and that he had never dissuaded him from taking any other treatment, orthodox or otherwise. All decisions as to therapy were to be Caron's alone. Having opted for 714-X treatment, Caron went back to the surgeon to tell him of his decision, only to be insultingly told to his face that he was "off his rocker"!

Caron began a series of twenty-one injections, which was repeated three times running, for an overall total of sixty-three. Because his salesman's job required extensive travel throughout Canada, some of the injections into his lymph node were substituted, as a stop-gap measure, for applications of the product with a swab directly under his tongue.

Then Caron got to the "punch line" of his story. Sixty-five days after the 714-X treatment had begun, declining to return to the hospital where he had been insulted by the surgeon, Caron had his medical file transferred to Montréal's Victoria Hospital, where he asked specialists to perform on him every conceivable test to see whether there was any cancer left in his body. Following the tests, he was told that he was completely free of the disease. That was in 1982, and Caron remained in perfect health up to 1988, when he began to suffer from pain in his left hip. Fearing his cancer might have returned, he had three more weeks of tests made, only to be told there was still no trace of any cancer present and that he had contracted a case of what is known as Paget's disease.

In his conclusion, Caron made clear that he had come to testify not solely about his own recovery from cancer. "I am not here to defend alternative medicine against traditional medicine," he affirmed, "but to say that I, and all other people, should be granted the right to choose the treatment we see fit." And, lest the jury might have missed the point, he added that one only had to compare his recovery with the demise of his younger brother.

There was no cross-examination of the witness.

Caron's testimony, no more, but certainly no less, impressive than any of those preceding it, was followed by an account so gripping in all its detail that it might well have upstaged all the others presented up to that point in the trial. The account was delivered by a lanky Belgian-born professional translator and interpreter, Arnault de Kerckhove Varent, whose craggily handsome visage was made all the more so by one obviously dysfunctional eye.

Launching into his own tale of woe, Varent told how, in the late 1970s, he had been diagnosed—like Claire Nuer— with a melanoma of the eye. And, just as in Nuer's case, cancer surgeons had recommended what technically is known as an "enucleation": cutting the eyeball out of its socket. Less than enthusiastic, Varent asked what he could expect, by way of survival time, if he refused the operation.

"Nine to twelve months," he was told.

"And if I submit to it?" he asked.

"Then you begin to *pray!*" was the only reply.

That was more than enough for Varent. After categoric refusal to take the orthodox medical advice, he instead decided to seek what he called "systemic" treatment that would affect not just the site of the tumor, but the whole of his bodily system. He and his relatives began making calls to Great Britain, Ireland, the rest of Europe, and the United States in search of such a therapy. At last, by telephoned word of mouth, they heard, through Stephen Zalac, the same man who had taken it to Vera Cruz, in Mexico, about Naessens's product.

Varent traveled to the port city on the Gulf of Mexico, where, at the Andrade Clinic, he was injected intralymphatically with 714-X, already being used experimentally in Mexico before it ever had been put to use in Canada. Before administering the product to Varent himself, Dr. Andrade had eye specialist medical colleagues confirm the Canadian diagnosis of melanoma.

Varent's tumor was, as the Greek word *mela* denotes, "black" in color, but, after the first set of twenty-one injections, its ebon cells began to turn an amber color, suggesting that the body's immune system was destroying them in a natural way. After a second set of injections, the color became lighter still, implying that the melanoma cells were disappearing, or had completely disappeared. The Mexican doctors were astounded.

Having offered all this testimony in detail, Varent also reported in court that, subjectively speaking, after the first series of treatments had reached only its fifteenth day, he began to feel "a whole lot better" than he had for months.

Finished with treatment in the city of the "True Cross," Varent returned to Montréal to take up his work. From Mexico, he brought back enough of the product for two more series of twenty-one injections in case he should ever need them. Need them he did, due to an unforseeable incident. One evening, while hefting a heavy box in his cellar, Varent cracked his head on a door handle so forcibly that he almost lost consciousness. Following the incident, the pain he had earlier felt in his eye so surprisingly returned that he feared that the melanoma was resuming its growth.

Given this important part of Varent's testimony, it is equally important here to note that one of the ways the body's immune system can be subjected to sudden, unwarranted, and unwanted stress is through a sudden shock brought on by just such an accident as the one which Varent suffered.

On a more personal note, I can say that I had long wondered why a friend, successfully treated by 714-X for cancer, had suddenly relapsed, until it was finally revealed to me that she had been exposed to trauma, brought on by a precipitous fall. Entering an apartment in Rome, Italy, while in the process of successfully recovering from her disease, she had not seen three steps leading from its foyer down into its spacious living room because, with its blinds drawn, the whole apartment, unlit by any lamp, was nearly pitch-black. Dashing to open the blinds, she had catapulted over the stairway's edge to crash down onto the hard living room floor.

She fell so heavily that she was unable to get up and, subsequently, had to be taken on a stretcher to the airport and flown back in a sorry condition to the United States, where her immune system, unable to recover from the shock, permanently gave up its normal function of protecting the body from cancerous cellular development that, proceeding apace, finally led to her death. This story is told here only to illustrate how, as in the case of Varent's stunning, accidental trauma can play a disastrous role in the whole process of treating the immune system and, thus, the body as a whole. And it strongly suggests that patients undergoing such treatment must be far more careful to avoid accidents than those who do not require it.

After his second round of treatment, which, having learned to do so, Varent administered to himself, the linguist visited a physician friend in Ottawa who introduced him, in turn, to an eye specialist colleague. The second doctor, said

Varent, was "utterly flabbergasted" to learn that Varent had survived a diagnosis of eye melanoma for, by then, almost four years. "I simply can't believe it," he declared, "it's just not possible! You should have metastases all over your body, by now, right down to your big toes!" The physician was so dumbfounded that he asked Varent if he would consent to come to a special meeting of eye doctors. At the meeting, he sat on a chair in the middle of a room, his head covered to reveal only his affected eye, where every one of the some forty specialists assembled took a careful look at it. All agreed that they were witnesses to what amounted to an impossibility.

"You should have sold tickets to this show!" Varent joshingly ribbed the meeting's organizer, who, so perturbed that Varent's "cure" was simply "out of the question," warned him that, to be *really safe*, he should consent to an operation that would remove not only the eyeball but all the tissue around the empty socket.

Submitting to what was unrelenting pressure on the part of an orthodox eye physician whose medical beliefs simply could not tolerate the idea that 714-X could possibly result in a happy, and permanent, end to Varent's difficulties, Varent finally agreed to an "enucleation," the limited and less drastic form of surgery. At this point, the doctor, gloomily and threateningly, told him: "Well, if we proceed that way and remove only the eye, if all the rest of the tissue should prove cancerous, we may not be able to safely go in again and get it out."

Once again, Varent had had enough. "Just the 'enucleation,'" he said, sticking to his guns in the face of insistent and domineering "authority." Because of his refusal to take the advice proffered, he was then required, as was his wife and daughter, to formally sign an affidavit exempting and releasing the hospital and the doctor from all responsibility for him and his case, should matters turn out to be as bad as pessimistically predicted.

After the operation, the surgeon, again in open disbelief, said: "It's just incredible! None of the tissues around your eye had a single cancerous cell in them!" One would have thought that the doctor would have been, like his patient, overjoyed at this finding. Instead, he still continued stubbornly and persistently to insist that Varent just *had* to have metastases *somewhere* in his body. And, just as tirelessly, he also insisted that his patient undergo "prophylactic" radiation all around the eye socket, just to "make sure." Could there be any better example of the enslavement of orthodox medicine by the philosophy to which it is wedded?

Sick of the unrelenting pressure, Varent again resolutely refused the advice. He returned to Naessens's lab, where Naessens's microscopic analyses of his blood and urine came up with nothing but extremely positive results. Overjoyed, Varent nevertheless was subject to nagging doubt. "Because of the very *fear* instilled in me by doctors," he said, "and the 'negative thoughts' to which it gave rise, a few weeks later, I went back to the lab to have a second round of analyses. All were positive. *Even then,* I was not sure I was 'out of the woods,' so upset had I become by all the dire prognostications I had heard. So I gave myself another thirty injections of 714-X, after which a third set of analyses showed that my blood was absolutely 'clean.'" And he has returned every year since, with the same result, even though he has taken no more injections.

Varent's testimony was at an end. When Melançon had no questions to put him in "cross," the interpreter, like other witnesses before him, willingly made his whole medical file available to the prosecution. As he submitted the thick pile of documents to the court, Chapdelaine suddenly remembered that he had forgotten to request of Marcel Caron permission to do the same with his file. To correct the oversight, he called Caron back onto the stand. While offering his file for inspection, Caron said that he was *pleased* to do so if only because the file had been requested in a "polite and civil" manner, in contrast to the way it had been earlier sought for by agents from the Medical Corporation who had ransacked his house, in an attempt to find it, as if they were not appointed "police" officials, but just "thugs."

This aroused the ire of the prosecutor, who, for the first time, put a question to a defense patient-witness. With almost studied rudeness, he shot out at Caron: "They weren't really *police*, were they, now? Did they wear *badges*?" As if all "policing" roles, or "police"-type actions required such.

Shooting the prosecutor a withering look, the disgusted Caron said quietly, "What does it matter? Up to then, as a free law-abiding citizen, I'd never had anyone break into my house to search it!"

That put an end to the prosecutor's questioning and he collapsed back into his chair as if he had received, deservedly, at least a slap in the face, if not a blow to the jaw.

To relieve the appearance of witnesses dominated only by males, Chapdelaine next introduced Suzanne Berthiaume, a pertly attractive, petite, forty-year-old, curly-haired blonde. An employee of the Canadian federal government, Berthiaume said she had been diagnosed with breast cancer on 5 December 1988, and, like thousands of women similarly diagnosed, had been strongly advised to have the afflicted breast immediately cut off. Trying to recover from the shock of the pronouncement, she said she would go home and think about it the night through.

When Berthiaume returned to the hospital, she asked what treatment, if any, she would have to undergo after surgery, and was told that she would have to take doses of the same old "radiation and chemotherapy" to which thousands of cancer patients have been exposed, all over the world, at great cost, but with so few overall results.

Thinking about her father, who, after being diagnosed with lung cancer, had himself submitted to such "tried-and-true" ministrations, but who had subsequently gone on to die in great discomfort, Berthiaume firmly refused all standard treatments, a decision, she told the court, that caused the doctors milling around her to go into a "near panic."

As had others before her, the well-spoken Berthiaume was recommended to Naessens. After also being given no promise of cure, she took three sets of twenty-one injections of 714-X from 12 December 1988, or one week following the initial diagnosis, to the end of April 1989, or just about one month before Naessens's arrest and inculpation as a "charlatan" and a "quack."

"Since then," Berthiaume told the court, "I have had a tremendous feeling of well-being, even a renewed 'lust for life.' And when, at my own initiative, I went back to the clinic where I had first been diagnosed, for tests, I was told that I had no trace of cancer left in my body."

After getting Berthiaume to agree, like preceding patients, to make her medical dossier available to the court, Chapdelaine, looking at his adversary at the table opposite his own, said: "Your witness."

To which, once again, Melançon replied: "No questions."

If Berthiaume's concise acount of her recovery, I thought to myself, had not impressed the jury's men, it surely must have made an undeniable impression on its women, for, with all the propaganda circulated by medical orthodoxy about the necessity for women to have regular, or repeated, mammographies, which of the members of that sex is not daily constrained, however unwillingly, to consider that she might not, sooner or later, be put through the same trials and tribulations as the witness?

There were two more witnesses to go, the first of whom was already known, in that his appearance at an earlier summer press conference had already been reported in the July newspapers. This was Renaud Vignal, the French ambassador to the Seychelles. The commandingly distinguished diplomat's remarks to the court have already been reported, for the most part, in the first section of this book. What can be added here is that, as he stressed for the jury: "When I first went to see Naessens with my wife, Anne, I was skeptical, enough so to play the 'devil's advocate.'

"What caused me, almost on the spot, to abandon that role," added Vignal, "turned me completely around," were three things: (1) Naessens's "complete humility" with regard to his treatment, and his profound faith in its ability to reinforce the immune system; (2) the fact that Naessens advised Madame Vignal to keep on with the chemotherapy recommended to her, so as not to "burn any bridges behind her"; and (3) Naessens never once having asked of the Vignals, man or wife, for a single dollar—or penny—in fees.

Furthermore, said the diplomat, Gaston Naessens was the only person among the countless medical personages he and his spouse had consulted who, with respect both to her survival or to the possibility of their having a much-wanted child, had *"given us any hope at all."*

Asked by the prosecution whether he had told her doctors about his wife's 714-X treatment, Vignal replied that he had not, because neither of them had wished to cause the medical professionals any annoyance or embarrassment.

To the growing stack of medical files already presented to the court, Ambassador Vignal added that of his wife.

As his very last witness, Maître Chapdelaine called a man whose identity he, and the Naessenses, had taken great pains to conceal as the trial was progressing in order that, in light of his professional status, the full impact of his appearance and testimony might most strongly be felt by all at the trial. When the French ambassador stepped down and took his seat among the spectators, up to the witness stand walked a man whose white-bearded profile was a near copy of Sigmund Freud's. After taking the oath and being asked by the clerk to name his profession, François Wilhelmy replied with a single word: "Judge!"

At its pronouncement, one could have imagined that a bolt of lightning had struck the tiny room. That a judge of the court of the province of Québec had decided to appear on behalf of a defendant accused of a crime that, were he found culpable of it, might incarcerate him for life seemed most unlikely. Moreover, it surely must have imparted a general feeling that the whole weight of provincial justice and law was by no means solely directed to proving Naessens's criminality. Quite to the contrary, here was a senior representative of the legal system standing foursquare to uphold the notion that Naessens had done nothing wrong, and that there was "something rotten in Denmark," and in Québec, about a medical system that had forced him to offer a potentially life-saving method of treatment in clandestinity.

To summarize what Judge Wilhelmy said, we shall refer to Jacques Lemoine's report in the Sherbrooke *Tribune:*

The judge testified in favor of Naessens that he, and his wife, stricken with cancer, had consulted with the researcher *after* his arrest. The couple considers that his product, 714-X, represents the "only remaining life raft" for her salvation. In an astonishing deposition, he talked on behalf of his wife, who, having had her larynx surgically removed, was incapable of testifying out loud.

Married since 1952, and father of five children, one of them a doctor of medicine, he told how his wife had begun treatment in 1979, for a cancer which began to reappear in 1985. And in March 1989, he learned that, the cancer having become severely aggravated, there was no more treatment that could alleviate his wife's condition, with the exception of tranquillizers.

In July, the magistrate and his wife consulted Monsieur Naessens who agreed to help them. The judge said that it was no "charlatan" he had gone to see, but a true scientist.

"Madame Wilhelmy has now got much of her strength back," declared the Judge, "and, since getting the 714-X treatment, has been able to take up all her various activities."

That was the bare bones of the case. To which can be added that the judge also testified that Naessens had never made him or his wife any promises and that, after having taken three sets of twenty-one injections each, metastases visible on her neck had begun to recede.

When the prosecutor asked Wilhelmy who had performed the 714-X injections, the judge, looking at his peer on the bench, rather than at Melançon or the jury, answered: "I prefer not to answer that question, *Votre Seigneurie*! If, however, this tribunal requires that I must do so, I shall reveal the name. What I can and will say is that the person was neither Monsieur Naessens nor myself. The 'sub-rosa' treatments were administered at a location not far from our home."

Then, by way of conclusion, Wilhelmy, who put his wife's medical file on the pile already publicly made available, added what may have been the trial's strongest statement, strongest just because it came from no less a "Lordship" than Péloquin himself: "That such treatments, as Naessens's 714-X, are not publicly available is more than distressing. Why do they have to be hidden? After all, in our society, any of us would make any and all attempts to rescue, to save, a drowning man, woman or child . . . so why not a victim of cancer?"

None could have summed up the issue, central to the judicial proceedings, more succinctly. But nobody was there to give a reply to the question. And, with that, the defense rested its case.

When the jury was dismissed, the presiding judge allowed, to my utter surprise, a photographer to enter court and make photographs of Péloquin and any others present.

It seemed that the judge, in making a rare exception to the rule "No Photos in Court," had been motivated by his having been miffed that an artist's absurdly sketched caricature of him had been printed, the week before, in the *Journal de Montréal*, and Péloquin wanted the same tabloid to run a photo that would reveal him as he actually looked.

The suspension of the rule allowed me to snatch my own camera from my pocket and take photos all over the place. Just as I was taking my last shot, I felt a hand on my shoulder, and turned to see the usually sober-faced Jacques Lemoine smiling a little smile, and to hear him say, "You know, Monsieur Bird, I feel I should tell you that, in over a quarter-century of court reporting, I have never heard testimony as moving as that to which I have listened for the past three or four days." His statement, which caused me to brush away tears, seemed to bode nothing but good for Gaston Naessens.

When court resumed its proceedings, Maître Chapdelaine asked that he be allowed a day of recess to prepare his final plea, a request Judge Péloquin found "perfectly acceptable." The jury was called back to be told that it would have a "day's vacation," and that, the next day, they would hear final pleas, first from Chapdelaine, then from Melançon. "The day after that," added Péloquin, "I shall give you my own address, to summarize the trial and instruct you on *points of law*," after which "vous allez entrer en délibération."

As they rose to make their exit, I wondered whether the jurors, as they reflected upon the "deliberations" upon which they were about to "enter," would, in their hearts, also be echoing Jacques Lemoine's heartfelt comment to me.

The tide of the trial had now almost crested to its peak. Since I was falling behind on the task of setting down notes on its day-by-day proceedings, and wanted to catch up before its rising waters had reached their neap, I was more than glad that I would, like the jury, be afforded twenty-four hours of respite from court attendance, if not a day's "vacation." Sitting in my little "cell" in Le Baron Hotel, I was once again struck with admiration at how Chapdelaine, with as much measure as circumspection, had chosen his limited parade of witnesses, each one of whose backgrounds had been carefully selected to coordinate, and to contrast, with those of all the others. For, had he wished, Chapdelaine could have called other witnesses, even from among spectators in the courtroom, such as Sylvie Corriveau, a young woman in her twenties, who, due to 714-X, has all but recovered from a serious case of multiple sclerosis.

Or, from among other Québécois notables, known far and wide throughout the province for their professional attainments, he could have called Normand Hudon, a celebrated caricaturist, cartoonist, and painter. While the trial was in session, Hudon was featured in the 4 November 1989 issue of *Échos-Vedettes*, under a headline taken from words he had spoken during an interview: "L'attitude du Collège des Médecins est écoeurante!* Le Dr Naessens m'a sauvé du cancer." "Docteur Naessens Saved Me From Cancer." "The Attitude of the Medical College Is Sickening!" "Sickening" rather than "Health Giving"—how could a better word have been found to describe it?

In the article, Hudon stated that he had been astonished that, as the trial was moving along its way, he had not been besieged by the media about "my surprising return to health after my receiving injections from Gaston Naessens." "I had prostate cancer," added Hudon, "as I was told in a Sherbrooke hospital a few years ago. But five months later, after the Naessens treatment, I went back to the same hospital, where it was declared by doctors that I had no trace of cancer left. None of them could understand it!" To cap his remarks about how well he had since felt, Hudon told the journalist interviewer: "You can say that I'm 'farting fire!'"

Écoeurante, in French, literally means "heart removing."

To anyone who sat, as I did, musing about what the opposing attorneys would bring out in their final pleas, two anal-
ogies might have comparatively come to mind. On the one
hand, the whole thrust of Melançon's "proof" had been made
up, as it were, only of a long series of stabs, as desperate as
they were misaimed. On the other, the totality of Chapdelaine's
presentation, with its masterful assembly of witnesses—not
too many, but "just enough"—seemed to have produced the
effect of a battering ram, inexorably striking its target, over
and over again, in exactly the same, and intended, spot. My
overall conclusion was: How could the defense possibly fail
to win this case?

Yet, like many others, I wondered whether the prosecutor, who was to present his plea following that of Chapdelaine's, might not, by his being able to leave the jury with
its last impression, have a tremendous advantage.

When, on the 29th of November, the judge and jury had
taken their places and all the rest of us finally were seated,
there was an almost "crackling" quality in the atmosphere,
made tangible by a single glance at the tense anticipation of
the defendant and his wife, as reflected on their faces when
their legal champion rose to address the jury.

Chapdelaine's introductory remarks were accented, above
all, with politeness. To the jury, he offered his profound
thanks, for their consistent "patience and attention." To the
judge, he offered his respect for a "tolerance and strong sense
of justice" exhibited over the years and, now, "over the past
three weeks, on behalf of Gaston Naessens." Finally, to his
adversary, Melançon, he proffered congratulations for "ably
playing his prosecutor's role in a difficult case, a role that,
having been assigned to it, he had no option other than to
accept."

Lowering, rather than raising, his voice for emphasis,
the defense attorney, whose gracious opening had served to
set everyone in the courtroom at their ease, looked squarely

at the jurors, all of whom returned his fixed gaze, to remind them, not of what Naessens was accused, but of what he was *not* accused, though he might have been. Specifically: any "illegal practice of medicine," or "concocting an illegal medicinal," that is, one without a federal *certificat de conformité.*

It was, he next cautioned the jurors, up to the Crown to convince them, in its own final plea, that "the accused had, through his representations or actions, actually caused the death of a cancer victim." But not that alone. They must, he warned, also be convinced that any "promise of cure" purportedly made by the defendant was a "knowingly false one" and, additionally, that it had been made with an "insouciance déréglée et téméraire" (an immoderate and reckless lack of concern) for her well-being.

"Si vous voulez" (if you will)—his polite tone had returned—"let us go over, once again, the whole story of Madame Langlais." Whereupon, he then, step by step, statement by statement, and fact by fact, covered every thing of significance that Dr. Lorenzo Haché had stated, or misstated.

It would be pointless, in this account, to set down every detail of the plea, but we might note here that, in order to make it crystal clear to the jury that it was indeed a ticklish matter to decide whether a cancer patient's tumor had so metastasized as to assure the impossibility of survival, Chapdelaine referred to a recent cancer-induced death of a Québecer, Jean-Claude Malépart, well known to the province's whole population, due to his elevation to the rank of a member of Parliament. Noting that, whereas no metastases had been found in the minister's body after his original cancer tumor had been detected, a second tumor, that sped him on the way to the grave, had also appeared, indicating that, though undetectable by any known test, metastases had indeed been present.

The defense attorney's use of a case pertaining to a political figure as familiar as Malépart seemed to dispose of the whole question, laboriously discussed in the trial itself, as to whether metastases could or could not have existed in Madame Langlais's own body and thus doomed her, even before she went to Naessens for consultation. As Chapdelaine concisely put it: "Thus, tests that 'find nothing' also 'prove nothing.'" And to nail down his argument, he also went over the pathologist's affirmation that the autopsy of Langlais had confirmed that she had the most aggressive cancer cells in her from the very outset, "undifferentiated" cells, which, once they begin to proliferate, never alter their nature.

Turning to the prosecution's main thesis that, in making her a "knowingly false promise" of cure, Naessens had prevented her from possible cure at a hospital, through surgery and other conventional treatment, Chapdelaine made a number of points. First, witness Sisso had repeatedly referred to her "fear" of hospitals, operations, and, in fact, the whole of orthodox medicine. Second, her decision to opt for Naessens's 714-X treatment was hardly "strange" when one considered that other cancer afflictees, such as Caty, Wallaczek, and Berthiaume, refusing to go the operative and chemotherapeutic route, had also opted for the same treatment. As also had Caron, who knew enough not to follow in the tracks of his brother. That Langlais had "unreasonably" refused traditional treatment, as Melançon was alleging, itself seemed unreasonable, stated Chapdelaine, inasmuch as the witnesses he had just cited had done so entirely "reasonably."

Third, asked Chapdelaine: "How can Naessens possibly be held to have promised Langlais a 'cure' when he had promised no such thing to Gary Diamond, who was visiting his laboratory at approximately the *very same time* as she was visiting it?" Nor, he added, had Naessens promised "cures" to Wallaczek, Caron, or Judge Wilhelmy and his wife. "In fact," he declaimed, "*none* of the witnesses who took 714-X injections, and got better, not *one* of them, was ever promised a 'cure'! All they were told by Naessens was that his product might well strengthen their immune systems. All my witnesses, *without exception*, said this very same thing! So it seems that Monsieur Melançon is clearly wrong in affirming that my client said the very opposite to Madame Langlais!"

As to the claims of expert prosecution witnesses Carter and Jasmin that 714-X was ineffective with regard to cows, dogs, or even rats, "why, then," asked Chapdelaine, "why on earth, has it worked successfully on humans, as Michel Fabre, a doctor of medicine, has clearly attested? Worked on such patients as Claire Nuer, whose eye melanoma, one of the most virulent of cancer forms, had been arrested? Or, for that matter, on Arnault de Kerckhove Varent, stricken with the same affliction? And even worked on one of the Crown's own witnesses, Roland Caty?"

Melançon, went on Chapdelaine, had referred to the patients' cures being "all in their minds," to a "placebo" effect, and thus intimated that those phenomena alone were responsible for their betterment rather than a product that "experts" had shown was "utterly worthless." If that were so, he continued, "then how come a senior judge of the Québec court has told you it allowed his own wife to virtually come back to life from death's door?" "Think about these things," he said soberly. "If you do, you will see that it's not necessary to know exactly what ingredients are in the 714-X product. When you think about patients, who had been condemned and abandoned by orthodox medicine, such as Jacques Viens, who was sent home to die, *what more is needed?*"

Furthermore, noted the defense attorney, there was something extremely *gênant*, extremely "troubling," about the fact that, of all the medical dossiers seized by Grégoire and his search party, only two were retained and some 148 more returned to Naessens. "Could it have been because all, or most of them, instead of providing any evidence of malfeasance on Naessens's part, contained proofs of cure such as is provided by all the dossiers already made available to

this court? And don't you think that it's more than strange
that the medical authorities, who have been able to have a
look at them, have paid not the slightest heed to the positive results they set forth?"

Building his solid defensive wall, brick by brick, Chapdelaine did not stop there. Sweeping wider so as to bring out
the real enormity and monstrosity of the trial's central issue,
he asked, "How is it that an individual, biologically trained,
researcher has been so virulently attacked by the medical
profession when his discoveries have been heralded, and
lauded, by such men as Michel Fabre, one of its own members, and by Rolf Wieland, a microscopy expert for the world-
known optical firm Carl Zeiss, whose letter sent in September of this year, attests to the uniqueness of his microscope
through which even prosecution witness Dr. Yvan Boivin said
he had seen a 'whole new world'?" The question was a stirring one, but Chapdelaine could not offer an answer, as we
have done with citations from Beverly Rubik's article. But
the rank unfairness, in the heart of that question, cannot but
have caused the jurors to ponder and reflect.

Chapdelaine was nearing his conclusion, mortaring the
final bricks onto his wall. "You see, there *are* approaches in
medicine, other than the orthodox one, approaches discovered by geniuses such as Naessens! Dr. Fabre has clearly
shown you that Naessens's approach is not one of spraying
a few mosquitoes with pesticides, but of getting rid of the
whole swamp in which they continue to proliferate. Dr. Haché
referred to 'marginal' techniques in medicine. But why should
a technique, such as Naessens's, an exceptional technique,
to be sure, be castigated as 'marginal'? If such techniques are
so castigated, then how are brand new discoveries *ever* to be
recognized for what they are, that is, salutary . . . *life saving*?"

The key to what Naessens had developed, stressed Chapdelaine, was his approach not to eradicating cancer cells *artificially*, as was everywhere attempted by orthodox cancerology,

but to assisting the immune system to do so *naturally*. "If this is successful, as we have proved it is," he added pointedly, "then how come members of the Medical Corporation are not more open to it? How come? They are not only not open to it, not only not interested in it, but even stoop to attack those who have been successfully treated, however clandestinely, in this manner! A judge, Monsieur Wilhelmy, has told you how unfortunate it is that the treatment has to be sought out in so clandestine a manner. Does this not imply there's something legally askew?" The wall was getting higher and higher, but Maître Chapdelaine had not yet built it to its top.

"Why are patients, successfully given this treatment, harassed when the treatment itself, and their names, become known to the medical authorities? Why are dossiers on their medical histories, revealing the success of such treatment, cast on 'a garbage heap,' if you will, while experiments on dogs or rats are upheld as the whole truth of the matter? What we are dealing with here may be as fundamentally good an approach as seen in this century! Do we have to wait until the next century to see it approved? There's something totally incomprehensible going on here! Incomprehensibly inhumane! Millions and millions have been spent in cancer research over the years. Thousands and thousands of terminal cases have been told things are 'hopeless.' Yet, what Judge Wilhelmy called an 'ultimate salvation' is not allowed them! Gaston Naessens can provide and has provided that salvation. And, now, he's not in his laboratory, but in a courtroom. It's just hard to fathom how our society can brook such intolerance!" The wall was up, to its full commanding height. It only remained for Chapdelaine to lay in the final brick.

"I ask you for acquittal"—it was a demand, rather than a plea—"on all counts. For, in reaching such a decision, you may be helping thousands who believe a new approach in medicine is necessary."

Chapter 11
"En Dehors de Tout Doute Raisonnable"

Naessens, a French-born biologist, may well be the most important figure since his countryman, Louis Pasteur, many of whose conclusions are upset by Naessens's research.
The Montréal Downtowner, 30 August 1990

It was an outstanding performance, a masterful address, one that, had it followed, rather than preceded, whatever prosecutor Melançon was about to say, would most certainly have produced the requested verdict of acquittal. Yet, before that verdict could be so pronounced, we, all of us in the courtroom, and especially the jurors, the ultimate "arbiters of truth," would have to listen to the prosecutor's final counterplea, which because it was time for the lunch-hour break, would be delivered in the afternoon.

It might be surmised that, while waiting for it to take place, Gaston and Françoise Naessens would have eaten their meal with little appetite, if they ate it at all. I do not know whether this was the case or not, because I did not share their table. I could, therefore, not tell whether they awaited Melançon's closing remarks with anxiety, or whether they believed that he might rupture the wall Chapdelaine had erected, or crumble it in its entirety, and thus ultimately deter the jurors from acquiescing to Chapdelaine's ringing request. I did not, could not, know anything about that until just this moment, as I am finishing my typing of this sentence.

So, I stopped the typing and called the Naessenses' Rock Forest number and, when Françoise answered the telephone,

I asked, "Did you eat your lunch with appetite, while waiting for Melançon's reply to Conrad Chapdelaine?"

Françoise chortled. "I think we did," she replied. "I also believe I know why you're asking the question. You want to know whether we had faith in the idea that our legal counselor's plea would bring Gaston the acquittal requested. Well, Christopher, we had *complete faith* that Conrad had done a superb job with his final plea, that no one in his shoes could have done a better one. Yes, now that I think back on it, we did enjoy our lunch." Of course, only the Naessenses, who had spent dozens of hours in consultation with Chapdelaine, could surely have had so abiding a confidence. In the King's Hall pub, across the street, where a band of us spectators, including two of Françoise's sons, were having our own lunch, the mood was less confident, more somber. The more pessimistic among us might be imagining Conrad's wall to be delapidating, even as we ate.

Promptly at 2:30 P.M., when court went back into session, the prosecutor rose. "I'm not going to detain you for long," he began, "I'm going to make it *'short and sweet'*"—he actually inserted those English words into the otherwise wholly French flow of his discourse—"and cut right to the heart of the matter."

That "heart," it turned out, was Melançon's main obsession that, as unbelievable as it may seem to others, patients faced with death by cancer are, if only out of fear of that death, capable of acting irrationally. To explain what he meant, the prosecutor said that he would put forward a theory that he himself had elaborated. "It's a theory based on a 'switch,'" he said, "you know, as in 'On . . . Off.'" Normally, reasonable people had their mental switches "On," but, once afflicted with cancer, their fear turned those switches "Off."

Having disposed, for the moment, of that psychological leitmotif, which he would nevertheless reintroduce as his counterplea proceeded, he next said that, while it seemed

that Chapdelaine had done his best to impress the jury with
Naessens's so-called accomplishments, all of the testimony
they had heard on that score was basically irrelevant to the
trial's central accusation, as explained by him at its opening—
that "Naessens had lied, and *knew* he was lying," when he
made Madame Langlais a promise of cure.

Melançon also made much of the fact that a Canadian
government laboratory chemist had said that Naessens's
product, 714-X, was no more than a tiny bit of camphor in
an aqueous solution. He again went over the statistical "numbers game," to try to convince the jury that Langlais would
have had a thirty-five percent chance of survival had she not
been dissuaded from undergoing Haché's surgery, plus further traditional treatment. He insisted that Dr. Haché had
unequivocally affirmed that 714-X was in no way useful for
treating cancer and repeated his statement that only "marginal"
doctors—those on the "lunatic fringe" was the implication—
ever used medicinals either unlicensed by the authorities or
unknown to the medical profession as a whole.

"You heard Dr. Haché clearly say," he intoned to the
jurors, "that if a medicinal was at all effective, then doctors
everywhere would know about it." And he also said that
"what's known is used," and "what's important to us is applied."

Sarcastically, Melançon further went on to state that,
not only did Naessens manipulate patients by telling them
what they wanted to hear, but that, by casting his defendant-
client in "humanitarian" guise, Chapdelaine had defiled a
humaneness common to all doctors.

Then, in a main thrust: "This trial is not being held to
assess the merits of orthodox, as against alternative, medicine." But, oddly, he didn't follow this up. There was no second punch to complement the first. Instead, he returned to
his "placebo" and "psychological suggestion" argument, but
weakened it when, after adjusting his glasses, he began referring to his handwritten notes to get his wording straight, just

as if, unsure of his argument, he was constrained to take it from a textbook.

Turning back to his "switch" theory, he next said to the jury: "Put yourself in the shoes of Madame Langlais! What would you have done? That promise of Naessens's would have been enough to turn your own, or anyone's, 'mental switches' off, as it obviously did hers."

In fact, it had been quite the opposite, I thought, in the case of one of my close friends, who, stricken with inoperable liver cancer, had resisted my advice to try Naessens's 714-X treatment, resisted it to the end, just because he had not turned *off* a "switch" that, while on, powered him with the prejudiced belief that such treatment could not possibly work, just because, as Haché had said, if it could, and did, it would be "widely known."

About Roland Caty's refusal to have his genitals surgically ablated, Melançon was sarcastic. "Maybe he was right on that, I don't know. Perhaps he had no metastases, wasn't as seriously afflicted as he was thought to be or, maybe, who knows, he just had a strong enough immune system to cure the cancer?" The prosecutor was now obviously swinging wildly, if not actually "shooting into the woods."

On and on he went with his theme that desperate patients are prone to lose their reason. "Ils ne sont pas équilibrés"— "they're unbalanced"—and it was due to that lack of equilibrium that Naessens was able to provide them with false hope. "That alone," he added, "allows you to understand why a lot of patients act so 'crazily,' so much so as to refuse normal treatment for cancer!"

Referring to Ronald Carter's failed experiments with dogs and cows, again, sarcastically, he commented: "Could it be that the animals treated with 714-X had *no confidence* in Carter? If it didn't work in scientifically controlled tests on animals, then how could it possibly work on people?"

Grasping at straws to keep himself, and his argument,

afloat, he noted that since several of the patients, such as Gary Diamond, who had testified to getting well via 714-X treatment, had taken not only the Naessens product, but *also* chemotherapy, it "was most likely that the latter, rather than the former, medicinal had effected their cures."

If, in that regard, the jury still remembered the eloquent testimony of Gary Diamond, I thought, they must have wondered who was now "switched off," if not Melançon. Worst of all, the prosecutor *wandered,* back and forth along the disorganized lines of his argument.

Attacking Dr. Michel Fabre and his testimony, Melançon resorted to caricaturing the physician as a "smiling little man dabbling in all kinds of therapy, 'musical,' and God knows what else." "Obviously," he added, "he was overawed by Gaston Naessens! Overawed by his theory about the 'somatid,' and its being the 'basis for life.' I don't understand all that, but that's what you were told. Well, people are allowed their opinions in a free country, such as ours, but that doesn't mean we have to open the doors to *anarchy,* medical anarchy or any other kind. We have *laws* for protection of the entire citizenry, laws which we either obey, or we don't. And those who do not obey them"—the reference was, of course, to Gaston Naessens—"must bear the consequences."

Melançon next went on to say that there had been a lot, far too much, talk at the trial about "collaboration" between Naessens and orthodox medicine. "Well," he said, "if that's what's wanted, let Naessens do as others do. La médecine orthodoxe n'est pas si bornée que ça! Elle a un esprit ouvert!"

But just the opposite had been borne in on the jurors by all of Chapdelaine's defense witnesses: Orthodox medicine was "as narrow-minded as that." It was *not* "open-minded."

It was to Melançon's great credit that, at this point in his remarks, he looked at the jury to ask: "You may wonder why I had no questions for most of the defense witnesses who claimed cure, or remission, of their cancers while on the stand!" And the answer to this question that he provided is of credit to him as well: "It's not the business of lawyers to overharass people like them. They made their choice." But then: "What is it I am trying to do? Certainly we are not putting alternative medicine to trial here. Nor are we putting 714-X on trial. What's on trial is a man . . . Gaston Naessens."

Melançon had, by now, clearly lost the threads in the weft and warp of his arguments. Instead of capitalizing on his point that Naessens had intentionally contributed to the death of a patient, back he went to matters concerned with, shall we say, whether "faith" can "heal." "Wallaczek, Diamond, and most of the other patients you heard testify," he said, "had *faith* that 714-X could cure them. Faith can 'move mountains,' we've all heard that! Madame Berthiaume had that faith! We don't really know what we're doing when we get cancer. With Ambassador Vignal, and his wife, it was the same thing. He became impressed with Naessens, even though he went to the biologist's laboratory prepared to be a 'devil's advocate.' And even Judge Wilhelmy said his wife had 'confidence' in her being able to be helped by Naessens's treatment."

Had I been a member of the jury, I would, by now, have wondered: What point is he trying to make? What's wrong with "faith" or "confidence"?

But groping as he was, Melançon kept plunging ahead, and backward: The animals treated in the experiments had no beneficial effects . . . and we know why . . . because the product is mainly *water*, with only a trace of camphor in it. Would anyone in his right mind inject *water* into a human cancer victim, if it didn't work with animals? Dr. Haché told you it was "worthless." Patient Caron said he could "put it under his tongue" just as well as inject it in his groin." "Well," triumphed Melançon, "it seems that 'anything at all' can help, even 'An Apple a Day.'"

Given all this rhetoric, it was again admirable on Melançon's part, that, once more, he admitted: "I have a lot of sympathy for the defense-witness cancer victims . . . don't get me wrong on that! That's why I posed them no questions in cross-examination. . . . They had, and have, hope. And I, myself, am humane enough not to try to take it away from them."

A humane action on his own part, for which, as we shall see, he would be taken to task by Augustin Roy, M.D., the president of the Québec Professional Corporation of Physicians.

Melançon's argument was nearly at an end. Trying to defend orthodox cancer-cure methods, he likened the situation to a good meal, prepared for children. "Objectively speaking," there was absolutely nothing wrong with the meal. But if one kid didn't like it, then his reaction was "subjective." But that did not mean that the meal *wasn't* good. Exactly the same analogy, he concluded, could apply to all the defense witnesses. Why could it apply? Though he did not spell it out, Melançon surely meant that the cancer victims paraded by Chapdelaine were no more than children who sulkily had refused to eat the "good meal" prepared for them by the "cut, burn, or poison" bunch.

"So you must decide the *truth* of the matter," Melançon concluded for the jury. "You must decide whether witnesses for the defense did *not* tell the truth, voluntarily, or involuntarily. There are always two sides to any coin, an objective, and a subjective, side.

"It's the same for the coin that is 714-X. Does it actually work through the lymph system, or is it a *placebo* that takes its effect through the *mind*? Or can it work, too, just under the tongue? I don't know. But you have to ask yourselves those questions.

"For you are now in charge of things. And in your deliberations, you must include whether you think Naessens was 'peddling *despair*,' abusing people's confidence. Madame Langlais had confidence in Naessens's product . . . but she died. So as you go about deciding whether he is innocent or guilty, do not fail to contemplate that." Prosecutor Melançon's wall-bashing attempt had come to its end.

The following morning (30 November 1989), just before the judge began his five-hour address, the court was virtually rocked by the appearance, as seemingly impromptu as it was sudden, of a shortish, balding man in a cardigan and a European-style student cap. Had the trial been taking place somewhere in the United States, the effect of his presence on spectators would have equaled that produced by the arrival of a Frank Sinatra or a Burl Ives in support of a defendant.

As the *Journal de Montréal* headlined the following day: "Gilles Vigneault to the Rescue of Naessens." Known widely in Québec, and in France, as the province's most celebrated chansonnier and bard, Vigneault's composition of songs such as "My country is not a country, it's the winter . . . my garden is not a garden, it's the snow!" has, over a quarter of a century, stirred an ethnic, even nationalistic, pride of homeland in a population that had, over its history, been so downtrodden by its "Anglo" rulers that the number plates on all its vehicles carry the understatedly bitter slogan: *Je me souviens* (I remember).

For nearly an hour, during the lunch break, part of which he spent strolling arm in arm with Gaston and Françoise Naessens through the hallways, Vigneault was interviewed in the Palais de Justice's second-floor corridor, right outside the courtroom, by a flock of press, radio, and television journalists as avid to take down his words as had he been a prime minister or a monarch.

The chansonnier explained that, though tired and "jet-lagged" by an overnight flight from France, where he had been on tour, he had decided, because of the urgency of Gaston Naessens's plight, about which he had been informed by Ambassador Vignal, to immediately drive to the Sherbrooke courthouse. "My chief reason for coming," he declared, "is to offer my support to Naessens, because what's happening here concerns, and is for the good of, all humanity, for the good of all people, anywhere, who seek hope while often being offered only despair."

The *Journal* movingly reported that it would have taken very little more impetus for the crowd to begin singing "Mon cher Gaston," in reference to a song that, sung on festive occasions, in tribute to anyone, was originally composed by Vigneault himself and first sung by the poet to greet Québec's beloved premier, René Lévesque, upon his return from France after a visit with General de Gaulle. Since then, it has become as well known in Québec as, say, the more banal "For He's a Jolly Good Fellow" is known throughout the English-speaking world. Had the words of the song actually been sung, they would have run:

Mon cher Gaston, c'est à ton tour
De te laisser parler d'amour!

(Our dear Gaston, your turn has come
to let yourself hear our words of love!)

Vigneault laid it right on the line when he characterized Naessens, who, as he made plain, had his "unconditional support," as no more than the victim of a "witch hunt."

The chansonnier repeatedly referred to the benefits of alternative medicine in general, and homeopathy in particular, since the latter treatment had brought his mother—nearly ninety-eight years of age—back to health after she had suffered horribly from osteoporosis (decalcification of the bones), after orthodox medical practitioners had ruled that her affliction, brought on by old age, was untreatable.

In closing his extended remarks, Vigneault sternly concluded: "One must seek, on humanity's behalf, medical progress blocked by a pharmaceutical lobbyism that, together with that of arms mongers, is one of the world's most powerful."

What effect Vigneault's appearance in the courtroom, as the equivalent of a "nationally revered hero," or "legend in his own time," may have had on the jury, or the judge, was hard to assess. But its effect on all others present was overwhelming. At the invitation of Maître Chapdelaine, Vigneault took his seat in the section of the court reserved for supporters of the defendant.

From my notes:

7:30 A.M., 1 December 1989: The jury has been out since 4:00 P.M. yesterday. It deliberated, with a two-hour break for supper, until 9:00 P.M. last evening, and will continue these deliberations uninterruptedly until it reaches a conclusion. Everyone is on tenterhooks wondering how soon the fateful verdict will come in . . . and what it will be: *Coupable* or *non coupable.*

The judge's extensive summary of the trial in which he went over all its details, testimony by testimony, and fact by fact, represents, despite its length, as brilliantly concise an overview as can be imagined, to the point where anyone interested in retrospectively following the trial's proceedings would need only to read that summary's transcript.

In his legal instructions to the jurors, Judge Péloquin, in clear and measured language, began by saying that what had been on trial in his courtroom was *not* a form of alternative medicine, but a person accused by the Crown of having contributed to the death of a patient through criminal negligence by offering her a false promise of cure . . . and knowing it was false.

His introductory remarks, which seemed to support the thesis of the prosecutor, rather than that of the defense, set what could be characterized as an "ominous tone" with respect to the outcome. However, as he proceeded, the court's president also made crystal clear that, to convict Gaston Naessens on so serious a charge, each jury member would, in his or her conscience, have to pass through five *étapes,* to run a gauntlet of five "stages," leap five hurdles, one could say. Bidding the *jurés* to make careful notes, he slowly dictated, a few words at a time, what those five hurdles represented, while every member of the panel took them down verbatim.

"(1) You must be convinced [and the next six words were indeed awesome], *en dehors de tout doute raisonnable,* that when the patient first visited Naessens's Rock Forest laboratory, she had a reasonable chance for a complete cure of cancer through orthodox treatment, and you must weigh the testimonies of the prosecution's expert medical witnesses in that regard!

"(2) If you successfully pass that barrier, you must next be convinced [and the repetition vibrated like an outsized gong], *beyond all reasonable doubt,** that Gaston Naessens actually promised the patient and her husband that, with twenty-one injections of his product, 714-X, she would be completely cured of breast cancer with metastases to lymph nodes!

"(3) Then, if you are still convinced at stage two, you must proceed to stage three, where you next must be convinced [and, again, sonorously], *en dehors de tout doute raisonnable,* that the promise made was a false one and that the defendant knew, or was presumed to know, it to be false!

"(4) Even if you are convinced at stage three, you still have to address, at stage four, whether *beyond all reasonable doubt,* Naessens indeed showed an *insouci-*

---

*In law courts of the United States of America, the word "all" is omitted, to limit the phrase to a less impressive "beyond reasonable doubt."

ance déréglée et téméraire [an "immoderate and reckless lack of concern"] with regard to the patient's life!

"(5) Finally, you must also pass a fifth, and last, stage, during which you must become convinced . . . *beyond all reasonable doubt* . . . that it was truly the promise of false cure that kept the patient from accepting orthodox treatment!"

I must confess that, having never before heard instructions from a judge in court of law, and given the solemnity with which they were delivered, and considering the seriousness of the charge with its potential sentence of life imprisonment, I was profoundly impressed at the protection from any hasty decision offered to Gaston Naessens by the five barriers through which the jury must necessarily have to pass if, in the end, they were to arrive at a verdict of "Guilty." And the verb "to convince," or its reflexive "to become convinced"—from the Latin *convincere,* that alternately means "to refute," "to convict," and "to prove," or all three at once—seemed to take on powerful new meaning. The jurors, as it were, would have to be able to "refute" all doubt, in order to "prove" to themselves that they should "convict" the accused. And I wondered whether, in their deliberations, the jurors would ask of themselves what Judge Péloquin's "become convinced," five times repeated, meant in all its subtleties.

Yet, even at that point, the ruling magistrate had not finished. Once again, though slightly more briefly, he went over the stages, one by one, and five more times repeated the fateful words: *beyond all reasonable doubt.* Then came his final words: "So, if you can conclude you have passed all five stages, you must return the verdict: *Coupable!*"

That was it. The trial was over. It was now up to five men and six women to render justice. The *jurés,* "those sworn," retired to begin their deliberations.

Outside, in the corridor, Naessens, on the face of things, seemed encouraged. "They can't possibly get through every one of these five barriers," he murmured to a small band of well-wishers around him. Could he have been just "making the best" of things, "whistling in the dark"? For, a few moments later, he said to me, and to the *Tribune's* Jacques Lemoine: "It's really spooky to think that my whole destiny . . . my very fate . . . now lies in the hands of eleven unknown men and women who haven't, can't have, the slightest idea of what *really* is at issue here."

So, as I write these notes, early this cold December morning, the jury will continue to deliberate, no one can be sure for how long, or with what result.

At 8:00 A.M., Ralph Ireland came over from his crystal mine twenty miles away from here, in Bonsecours, where, last night, he performed a "crystal ceremony": implanting a "thought" in a limpidly pure rock of quartz, one of his most beautiful, and, via the same gem, directing that thought to the jury. Never would I have believed, or have hoped, that so "occult" a practice, really an "energized prayer" in its way, might be effective! And I was sure that, throughout the same night, all of their supporters, and the Naessenses themselves, had been offering up their own prayers.

Ralph was on the telephone with someone at the local television station when his interlocutor excitedly interrupted him with the good news: "Gaston Naessens has just been acquitted on all counts!" It was a few minutes past 10:00 A.M. So it had taken the jury, gone back to its task at 9:00 A.M., only a bare hour more to reach its decision.

Our euphoria was indescribable. We hugged each other for a long minute. Our only regret was to have missed the final scene—the jury's entry into the courtroom to announce its decision.

It was Françoise Naessens who described it for me. Enthroned on his bench, Judge Péloquin, addressing no more than a dozen spectators present, warned that, whatever the verdict, he would brook no demonstrative reaction to it in his court lest any outbreak of emotion betoken a sign of disrespect for the jury, which had taken an extremely important decision. Asking the marshall to call in the jurors, he instructed him to tell them that their verdict must be delivered, not in any global fashion, but count by count.

After the jurors were reseated, they were polled by name, just as if they were members of a military platoon formed up on a parade ground prior to an early morning exercise. As each of them heard his or her name called, each answered: *Présent!*

At the judge's question "Who will speak in your name?" a handsome middle-aged woman, the chief of personnel for a local branch of the Royal Bank of Canada, rose to acknowledge that function.

It was then the turn of the *greffier*, the court clerk, to ask: "Est-ce que tous les membres du jury sont d'accord sur le même verdict?"

"Oui!" answered the jury chair.

The moment of truth was at hand. "Quel est votre verdict concernant le chef numéro un?" asked the clerk, as Françoise and Gaston Naessens, their relatives, and the two adversary lawyers were sitting figuratively, if not literally, on the edge of their seats.

"Non coupable!" was the chair's reply, a reply that was repeated four more times in answer to the same question on the succeeding, less serious, counts.

Holding to the judge's instructions, Françoise Naessens sat silently weeping, her head bowed almost to her knees. As for Gaston Naessens, he told me that, as each "Not Guilty" decision rang through the courtroom, he felt as if five heavy stones placed on top of his body were, one by one, being removed. And even Maître Chapdelaine, sitting next to him, while under perfect control during the voicing of the first two pronouncements, could not help letting out his own audible little sigh of relief at the third.

When Ralph and I raced over to the courthouse to congratulate the Naessenses on their victory, we found they had already departed. But there was Maître Chapdelaine being interviewed in the corridor by several journalists. Before he even noticed our presence, we took him, Ralph from in front, I from behind, in a dual bear hug, and the little guy grinned from ear to ear.

The next day the *Journal de Montréal* went "all the way" for Naessens. Filling its front page, in full color, was Gaston's face, beaming with a smile, and a huge headline, in yellow block letters, reading: NAESSENS ACQUITTED!

In a sidebar was a tribute from ex-minister Gérald Godin, who, in an interview entitled "I Really Owed Him That," said he was overjoyed at the decision of the jury. "It's good news for the health of the Québec people," the "star witness," as he was called by the newspaper, exulted. "It's fantastic for Gaston Naessens, for all those people he's treating, and for all patients to come!" Declaring that he had been glad to testify for Naessens Godin said, "That was my duty and I did it. I felt I really owed him that!"

The *Journal*'s feature story on Naessens's acquittal was only sullied, in its triumph, by another sidebar with a headline reading, "It's Twenty-five Years Now That This Farce Has Continued." These were the words of Dr. Augustin Roy, who had the temerity to berate the Crown's prosecutor for having done a bad job. Characterizing the trial as "wholly incomplete," Roy lamented that Melançon had not, as he most certainly should have, "savagely cross-examined every one of the patients who had testified on Naessens's behalf!" As if patients recovered through "any means" should be recommended for such heartless treatment by a so-called "doctor" who had no means to help them!

Augustin Roy did not stop there. In his great dissatisfaction, he ironically added: "All the patients that testified simply don't know the difference between *feeling* healthy, and *being* healthy." And worse: "All of them should *stand at attention* or, more properly, *get down on their knees* to thank orthodox medicine for having kept them alive!"

When I read these words, the statement of Jean-Hubert Eggerman at the summer press conference echoed in my ears: "We're not living in Stalinist Russia, or Nazi Germany, after all! We're in Canada! When am I, and all the rest of us, going to win the right to be treated as we see fit?" And that is exactly what the trial of Gaston Naessens had gone far to decide.

Part Three
Aftermath of Victory

Chapter 12
Tug-of-War

I pleased nobody except the people I cured.
                    Paracelsus, as quoted in *The Healer's*
                    Art by John Michael Francis Camp

There is no doubt that the victory in court was as triumphant as any won in the long history of battles fought in the legal arena between the orthodox cancer monopoly and those offering approaches other than "cut, burn, and poison," or that it had gone far to recognize the right of the latter to serious consideration. But, how far? That was the question.

Any attempt to provide an answer begins with an account of what happened directly following Naessens's acquittal. And that answer also involves the likelihood that, in the protracted struggle to come, the scales will, indeed must, be tipped by the weight of *public pressure.*

The struggle, thus, might be characterized as a "tug-of-war," not just between two diametrically opposed forces pulling on both ends of a single rope, but one with a second rope attached to the first's midpoint on which "outside" forces can pull at an angle to assure an ultimate victory.

Two days after the trial's end, a first tug on that second rope came when the *Journal de Montréal* printed a second full-page cover photo of Gaston Naessens, and a heartrending headline: "Three Hundred Cancer Victims, in Tears, Beg for Naessens's Famous Serum."

The appeals had been phoned in to the offices of the Committee for the Defense of Gaston Naessens on Montréal's Christopher Columbus Street, which, since the summer of 1989, had taken similar calls from desperate men and women all over Canada, the United States, and other countries

172

as faraway as Hungary and Chile, Australia, and the Union of Soviet Socialist Republics.

"While we are able to export 714-X abroad," committee chairman Bernard Baril told reporters, "we are now really helpless to do anything for our fellow Canadian citizens here at home until the Federal Office for Health and Welfare responds to Gaston Naessens's letter to Prime Minister Brian Mulroney." The letter to which Baril referred was written a little more than two months before the trial began. "Having devoted forty years of my life to the welfare of society," it read, "and believing that competent authorities are acting in that same spirit, I see no reason why we cannot sit down and come to an agreement. Since the problem has now gone beyond the understanding of our reductionist professions, I believe we now have the opportunity to develop a far more noble and virtuous overview of the whole question of health."

Naessens proposed to Mulroney that he furnish, free of charge, sufficient quantities of his products necessary for the treatment of patients. "I ask, on behalf of participating physicians and all others associated with the treatments, to give me your assurance that they will not be penalized for having participated in this clinical experimentation. I stand ready to participate personally in the evaluations and counterevaluations in which each and every one will have a right to make a contribution and in which I should not be placed in a defensive position." Then, getting to the nub of his problem, Naessens added: "A state of necessity justifies these urgent measures, *even if it is very difficult for many to see what they have never been taught to look at.*"

Since no reply, or other reaction, to Naessens's appeal for a "round-table" discussion to set up the requested experimentation had been forthcoming, Baril stated that cancer victims, who viewed the Naessens treatment as their only hope, were now panicking. "This is hard for all of us to swallow," he stressed, "and it's why we're asking top medical scientists in this country to devote serious study to this urgent question." The panic stemmed from the Defense Committee's having to inform all callers that Naessens's legal advisers had told him it was "out of the question" that he take on any new patients in what Judge Wilhelmy had called "clandestinity," and thus reenter a vicious circle of illegality. Urgently awaited was the government's decision to accord legal status to Naessens's medical products.

Baril also informed the reporter that the attack on Naessens by the Medical Corporation was still relentlessly being pursued by its president, Augustin Roy, as reported in the *Journal*'s story on the acquittal. "Dozens of people have called our office to express their angry indignation about this," he said. "It's now up to Ottawa to get involved because we are credible people despite Roy's claims to the contrary."

Also pulling on that second rope in the public's behalf were two articles by senior, and highly respected, journalists.

The first, written in a show of "hometown solidarity," was an editorial by Jean Vigneault, editor-in-chief of the Sherbrooke *Tribune*. Printed in double the normal-size type on 6 December 1989, with reference to medical "Tsar" Augustin Roy, it bore the title "The Don Quixote of Doctors." "It was neither reserve nor moderation," it began,

> that could muffle Roy's tone when he learned of Naessens's acquittal. Not only did he inveigh against the biologist himself, but even against the Crown's prosecutor, to accuse him of ineptitude. His further stating that the prosecutor had "manipulated" defense witnesses, and not sufficiently *frightened* them, won for Roy a deservedly harsh reprimand from the Crown's own prosecutor-in-chief.

Vigneault suggested that, while it was Roy's prerogative to defend the corporate interest of doctors, he should be fulfilling that mission, not by casting himself in the role of a Don Quixote, but by adopting an attitude of proper regard, and respect, for all individuals, including researchers who are not necessarily charlatans just because they do not belong to the same club as mainstream doctors. "When Roy has the gall to say that defense witnesses at the trial don't know the difference between *feeling* well and *being* well," he continued, "if he's not kidding, he's certainly demonstrating that he hasn't the shoddiest knowledge about human beings faced with grave illness and death."

Noting that the trial had not proved that Naessens's 714-X was a sure cure for cancer, the editorialist nevertheless held that its inventor should "merit the *high respect*, if not of doctors, then of all the rest of us, for having brought so much solace to hundreds of sick persons by allowing them to feel much better during a particularly agonizing period of their lives." And in a succinctly and toughly worded *envoi*, he concluded: "For there are surely no more patients who have died following Naessens's treatment than the ones who have died following treatments by the colleagues of Augustin Roy."

Roy's own reply to Vigneault's editorial, printed three days after Christmas, indicated that the erstwhile practitioner of medicine, turned "top policing agent" for his profession, had been wholly unaffected by its contents. Castigating the editor for presenting mere "opinion" based on "wild interpretations," he accused him of addressing a subject of which he had "manifestly no knowledge." More rudely he added, "He should have kept his trap shut, rather than leading his readers into error." The rest of the reply was a carbon copy, or "broken record," of the same diatribe that Roy had delivered on McGill University's radio station, as earlier reported in this book, without a single new reflection, or insight, added to it. Once again revealing his determination not to look into the facts of the matter, he sarcastically concluded that "only a novel" could do justice to the "Naessens Affair." In that single reflection, Augustin Roy, perhaps more than he realized, could well have been right.

A second pithy editorial contribution came as an unexpected Christmas present from the pen of Ed Bantey, the Montréal *Gazette* columnist who, as we have already seen, had written a stirring piece in the summer of 1989.

Bantey's Christmas Eve column, entitled "Gaspar Is a Miracle That Modern Medicine Can't Explain," was illustrated with the fetching photo of nine-month-old Gaspar Vignal, son of the French ambassador who had testified at the trial. In addition to being chosen partly to correspond to the first three letters in "Gaston," wrote Bantey, the little boy's name was taken from that of one of the three Magi, or Wise Men, who had followed the star to Bethlehem for the birth of Jesus Christ. This was because the A.D. 1989 Gaspar had, like his 1 B.C. cognomen, "traveled a long way to see the light." (See Appendix C for the full text of Bantey's article.)

In what amounted to "season's greetings" to his readers, Bantey related that Gaspar's mother, "whose physical frailty was no match for an inner strength," had used 714-X and that only its use could explain the miraculous birth of her son, a birth that had upset unanimous predictions by medical experts that she was fated never to have a child.

"Official medicine still maintains 714-X is worthless," wrote Bantey. "Frankly, I don't know if it is or it isn't. Either as a *cure* for cancer or AIDS, which Naessens himself says it *isn't*, or as a weapon in the fight against degenerative disease, which he and some scientists say it is. What we *do* know, is that Anne Vignal is alive, Gaspar is a thriving twenty-pounder, and dozens of cancer and AIDS victims believe the product has reinforced their immune system."

Noting that Judge François Wilhelmy had testified that he found it unacceptable that official medicine would deny people access to 714-X as a last recourse, Bantey added the one-line paragraph: "He's right, of course."

Then, saying that Naessens had offered to submit 714-X to objective analysis by qualified doctors and scientists, he concluded: "It would be unconscionable to refuse that offer. Think of what it might mean to mankind if that study proved in any way positive."

The editorial momentum created by Vigneault and Bantey was accelerated in two issues of *Sept Jours*. Its year-end "Retro '89" special edition offered a month-by-month retrospective roundup of the year's most important events that had taken place throughout the world, across Canada, and in the province of Québec.

Forty pages displayed color photos of Salvador Dali, Japanese Emperor Hirohito, the Ayatollah Khomeini, and other notables who had passed on during the year, and extensive illustrated coverage recalled for readers such political upheavals as the massacre of Chinese students on Beijing's Tiananmen Square and environmental catastrophes such as the *Exxon Valdez* oil spill in Alaska and the California Bay Area's earthquake.

In the three-page spread for the month of December, along with portraits of the "Invincible Mike Tyson," the "Rolling Stones," and the celebrated gymnast Nadia Comaneci, who had just escaped from Romania, was one of a smiling Gaston Naessens, seated in a white laboratory smock in front of his microscope. Naessens's December acquittal was thus judged by the magazine's editors to be one of the year's most newsworthy "happenings."

In its first issue for the year 1990, which became available to readers on 5 January, *Sept Jours* in its "This Week's Documentary Feature" followed up with a four-page article: "Gaston Naessens, Genius or Charlatan?" The exclusive report, written by Paule Daudier, and illustrated with four more appealing photos of Naessens—the largest one occupying one-and-a-half pages—began by casting Naessens in the role of a "microscopic Galileo."

Referring to Pasteur's years-long battle to win acceptance for his theories on microbiology and vaccination against an "all-powerful medical establishment," the journalist asked, "Can Naessens be compared to his predecessor? History will decide!"

Then she asked the biologist: "Isn't it a bit simplistic to tell someone: 'You have a precancerous condition and I'll give you 714-X, and you'll recover from it'?"

"That's quite right," Naessens replied,

> but isn't prevention much easier than cure? Patients have come to me in states of fatigue, been treated, and begun to feel in tip-top shape again. I'm certain that many of them were precancerous. Obviously, there is no traditional way of verifying that. But we can point to cases of cancer which were substantiated by hospital tests, so that the conditions of patients could be compared before, and after, treatment. In any case, my theories differ completely from traditional ones. Conventionalists say that *cancer is a local affliction that becomes generalized.* I say: "Cancer is a *general systemic illness that becomes localized.*"

"How do you react to Dr. Augustin Roy's statement that the cancer-victim defense witnesses at your trial don't know the difference between *being well* and *feeling well*?" asked Daudier. "And to his remark: 'The patients who go to see Naessens only inspire pity in me'?"

"That depends on what you call 'feeling better,'" shot back Naessens. "Isn't that preferable to 'not being cured'? I know people who have 'felt better' since 1949, following my treatment. When a dozen people from all classes of society come to testify under oath in my favor, then, if 'experts' claim my product doesn't work on dogs, or rats, of what importance is that? And how were those animal tests performed? In Guelph,

Dr. Carter injected dogs weighing 15 kilos *intravenously* with a daily dose of 20 cc. of 714-X, when a normal daily dose for a human weighing 60 kilos is 0.5 cc., injected *intralymphatically*. So that kind of experimentation is just senseless."

"You're not going to try to continue to live in illegality, are you?" Daudier asked in conclusion.

"Absolutely not!" confirmed Naessens. He continued:

> I want absolutely to put an end to all that! By appealing to *legislative* bodies, for as long as we keep trying to appeal to medical authorities, we get nowhere. We have to win a special *legal* status. We have to press forward. I've been totally blocked in my research for five years now. I want to be able to make my contribution, not on my behalf because I'm getting old, but on behalf of everyone. We're going to keep up the fight. That fight has not ended . . . it's just beginning!

As encouraging, publicity-wise, as were all these sympathetic editorial initiatives, they seemed to pale in importance when, immediately following them, Gaston Naessens scored another knockout in the jurisprudential ring.

In May 1989, a second series of criminal charges were lodged against the biologist.

In a court hearing held on the morning of 8 January 1990, spectators and a covey of reporters were stunned to hear chief prosecutor Michel Pinard declare that the Crown, in a proceeding known by the Latin appellation *Nolle Prosequi* (Not to Be Prosecuted), had decided to abandon its accusations under article 579 of the Criminal Code that permits such a stay while not having to provide reasons, or motivations, for it. When the prosecutor stipulated an *arrêt des procédures*, the judge immediately countered: "Monsieur Naessens est libéré!" The announcement that Naessens was "free to go" produced a round of applause from his supporters.

Interviewed outside the courtroom by representatives of the media, the elated defense attorney, Conrad Chapdelaine, expressed the opinion that the *Ministère public,* as the prosecutor is also known, had taken his decision after a thorough reevaluation of his proof following Naessens's acquittal by a jury. Meaning that, in his eyes, the proof, legalistically, no longer had a leg to stand on.

"It's a wise position that the Crown has taken," added Chapdelaine. "I was expecting it, at least I hoped for it. Even so, it's a really wonderful surprise! I also hope that the president of the Medical Corporation will take as wise a position between now and the month of June."*

Chapdelaine's reference to the 1990 summer month was in connection with a third series of accusations, this time for the "illegal practice of medicine," that have been lodged by the Medical Corporation. These involve eighty-two counts, for which, if found guilty, Naessens could be subject to a fine ranging from $25,000 to $400,000.

It seems, at least at the time of this writing, that Augustin Roy is in no mood to take any decision as "wise" as that of the prosecutor-in-chief, or as "wise" as that hoped for by Chapdelaine. After Naessens's second exoneration in court, it was obvious that he was still fixedly determined to carry on his vendetta to the bitter end.

Speaking with a reporter for the Montréal *Gazette,* he vindictively commented that Naessens's release from all criminal charges would in no way alter his position on a man that he had no qualms about calling a charlatan. "There is

---

*A note of levity: When, just before the hearing, I met Claude Melançon, who had lost his legal battle in the long November trial, and asked him, before a crowd of spectators waiting for the courtroom to open, whether he would once again be Chapdelaine's adversary, he replied good-naturedly: "Oh, no! It's been decided that I'm a legal rooster who lost too many feathers during the last cockfight! There's a tougher rooster in there to take my place!"

no reason for us to withdraw those charges against Naessens," he added, "and it's too bad the government doesn't prevent this person from exploiting human misery."

What Roy did not reveal to the reporter was that he was no longer in the commanding position of being able, fully armed himself, to attack an unarmed adversary.

The following day, the Sherbrooke *Tribune* ran a story back-to-back with its front-page account of Naessens's second court victory, headlined: "Gaston Naessens Seeking $200,000 Dollars in Damages Against the Medical Corporation."* The "moral and exemplary" damages were claimed in a libel suit against both the corporation and Dr. Augustin Roy personally, as a direct result of Roy's reply to editor-in-chief Vigneault's editorial that had been printed in the Sherbrooke *Tribune*'s 28 December 1989 issue, and to his comment about "a farce having dragged on for twenty-five years" as provided in a side-bar in the *Journal de Montréal* issue that had reported the Naessens acquittal on its front page.

In the eyes of Naessens's civil lawyer, Martin Gauthier, Roy's allegations constituted "deliberate attacks" on the repu-tation of his client and on his right to consider himself not guilty in the wake of his acquittal. Gauthier's suit accused Roy of "having made statements, in a libelous, defamatory and contemptuous way," as well as having been motivated by *"a hatred surpassing any normal limit."* The corporation itself was accused on the basis of having done nothing to stop the diffusion of the statements made by its president, and of having taken no action in favor of their retraction.

---

*The total damages requested were actually $300,000, it having been decided that the previously considered $200,000 was not enough. A court decision on this may be postponed for months due to an huge "backlog" of civil cases remaining to be tried.

Chapter 13
Cracks in the Wall

I am going to fight no matter what they do, because I believe I'm doing the right thing. I believe that this is our obligation to the people. If you find something that's valuable, you must continue and I believe we've found something that may be able to save lives.

Stanislaw Burzynski, M.D., Ph.D.,
Burzynski Clinic, Houston, Texas

In addition to this bold counterattack, one indication that Naessens might have made initial, and important, progress in winning first skirmishes in his battle against Roy in the medical arena was his having received a summons to meet with Canadian health authorities in Ottawa. It appeared that, after his 1 December 1989 acquittal, they felt they could at last sit down around a table with him to discuss matters brought up in his letter to the Canadian prime minister.

At a 20 December 1989 two-hour meeting with Dr. Michèle Brill-Edwards, director of the Department of Emergency Drug Release, and three other health bureaucrats, Naessens, flanked by Françoise and lawyer Conrad Chapdelaine, opened proceedings with a brief overview of his discovery of the somatid, its polymorphic cycle, and how these related immunologically to his theory of degenerative disease.

He was cut short by Brill-Edwards, who said her department was in no way interested in listening to any exposé of a new treatment mode, or the theory and philosophy that had led to its development, simply because the matter did not fit with the concerns and responsibilities of her office.

Handing Brill-Edwards a copy of the bulletin about 714-X issued by her department on 2 June 1989 (see pp. 52–53), Naessens asked her whether her office had, in fact, been responsible for the gross misinformation it contained. By way of reply, one of her staffers, while admitting this responsibility, and recognizing the distortions of truth contained in the communiqué, made no outright apology for them but only tried to make the excuse that, since the text of the bulletin was somewhat "telegraphic," details might have been overlooked.

Attorney Chapdelaine forcibly insisted that the document included unacceptable statements that had led the medical community as well as the broader public into serious error, and added that he was surprised that a Canadian federal office could have been so "cavalier" about the matter.

In true bureaucratic fashion, Naessens was next presented with a thick stack of material representing regulations, or procedures, through which any new "drug" must pass before it can be accepted, and legalized. "God," said Françoise to me, while pointing to the mass of documents in her Rock Forest home, "it would take me, or you, three full days, maybe a week, to go through, and understand, them." Instead of making any summary of their contents, let us simply state that, in its publicity supplement "Research on New Drugs: A Costly and Long-Term Investment," the Canadian Industrial Association for Medicinals reports that, from the time of its discovery to its first being put on the market, any new medicinal has to go through a process lasting from nine to twelve years, at an estimated cost of up to twenty million dollars (Canadian)!

Naessens then introduced the principal object of his visit, the same one raised in his letter to the prime minister: a "pilot project" to test 714-X on cancer and AIDS patients. The upshot was that, before any such testing could get underway, the health office would have to be provided with meticulously prepared medical dossiers of patients to be treated so that they could be studied by the officials before testing began.

How long it might take one researcher and his wife, working alone, and without any stenographers, filing clerks, or other assistants—or the funds to employ them—to put together the requested material for a federal office staffed with hundreds of employees, might be anyone's guess. But, even if the necessary documentation were provided virtually "tomorrow morning," there is no guarantee that, given the ponderous lethargy with which Canadian health "machinery" grinds in the approval of new medicinals, action to test 714-X, and approve its use, would quickly take place.

Consider, for instance, that Canada saw its way clear to approve vaccination for marsh fever, a form of malaria, only after seventy-four of the world's countries had officially sanctioned its use, and, then, only after Canadian citizens working in Asia for Hydro-Québec, one of the world's largest electric power companies, had come down with the affliction. To cite the comment of one newspaper report: "Subsequently, Canadians traveling to regions where marsh fever is rife have been routinely vaccinated by a product long since recognized by medical communities in Europe, and elsewhere."

By the first week of January 1990, the Ottawa health ministry was jolted when, encouraged by Naessens's acquittal and the favorable media publicity engendered by it, physicians—not only in Québec but in Ontario—began to dun it for permission to try 714-X on their cancer patients.

"Already, eight doctors have obtained authorization to prescribe the medicinal to patients, and some twenty more, both specialists and practitioners of general medicine, are awaiting such authorization," Naessens smilingly informed the Sherbrooke *Tribune* reporter Jacques Lemoine on 8 January 1990, directly after his second court victory. "The authorizations are made for 'humanitarian' reasons under an 'Emergency Drug Release Act.' When the permission is granted, the doctor can get the 714-X directly from me or my associates. So it's clear that there are at least some doctors who understand

that, since my acquittal, Augustin Roy's allegations that led
to my accusations don't count for much."

All of which hardly caused Roy to relax his stance. In
an interview on an English-language Montréal radio station
the very same day, he announced, "I am utterly surprised that
Ottawa would authorize the administration of a drug about
which they don't know anything. They don't even know its
composition or the way it's made. They don't know if steps
have been made to eliminate toxic reactions. They don't know
about the efficacy of the drug. So I think it's just a way to
try to do away with the situation without working too hard."

Magnifying these comments, Roy, as reported next morning by the *Journal de Montréal*, snappishly stated, "There are
limits to such folly and to this macabre farce! Ottawa seems
to be fawning before pressure put on it by Naessens's friends
who, through subterfuge, have learned how to exploit loop-
holes in the law."

Thus, having earlier attacked the competence of his
home province's legal prosecution office, Roy was now attacking the probity of his country's top office in matters of
health. In so doing, he was completely ignoring evidence, submitted at the trial, that the product's composition had *indeed*
been analyzed, that its nontoxicity had *indeed* been proved,
and that its efficacy had *indeed* been demonstrated.

And, so it seemed, were certain Ottawa health authorities ignoring the evidence, at least if one could believe what
was reported in an article in Montréal's *La Presse*. "Ottawa
Knows Nothing About Naessens's 714-X" read the headline
of a story by François Forest, the twists and turns of which
could have made anyone wonder whether Naessens had ever
made a trip to the capital city. "We know absolutely nothing
about 714-X at the present time," Health Ministry spokesman Michel Cléroux was quoted as saying. Then, as if Naessens had not supplied Brill-Edwards's office with a complete
laboratory analysis of the product that revealed all details

about its many components, the spokesman added, "What is known is that it is only an aqueous solution of camphor." Was this merely a repetition of what had been reported in the communiqué and, if so, did it reveal that one tentacle of the Health Ministry octopus didn't know what the other tentacles were doing?

For still another aspect of Cléroux's remarks, one had to turn to a report that ran the following day in the Sherbrooke *Tribune*. Referring to the meeting held in Ottawa with Naessens and noting that Naessens had been given the stack of documents as described above, the spokesman concluded that the "ball was in his court." "It is not up to us, Health and Welfare," he stressed,

to analyze or to test a product, whatever it is. The person who seeks to make it official must himself obtain recognized and accredited scientific proofs to start the process leading to an official recognition of the substance. There are various well-defined stages to be followed.

And all this must be done at the cost of the individual seeking authorization. Up to now we have never received even an introduction to a scientific proof so, for us, 714-X is only camphor and water. And that's it.

The spokesman, of course, did not mention that the "cost" to which he had referred might easily run into millions of dollars. About this, Naessens commented to the *Tribune:*

To fulfill the demand, one would need a platoon of scientists, working in several specialties, to make the required analyses. I'm afraid I haven't the money for such exigencies. I don't operate a pharmaceutical company making millions in profits. But I'm not giving up. I've already sent them a twenty-two-page report on my research, with complete analysis of 714-X, made by spectrography and other means. And I'm going to flood them with more information. I'll soon be sending them medical files on patients treated with 714-X over the last five years. I'm doing my level best to satisfy their requirements but I can't do the impossible.

As for doctors who had been petitioning Ottawa for permission to use 714-X, Cléroux was reported in the *Journal* as saying: "Since December, most of them who asked us for information on this solution have actually canceled their requests for permission to use it when we informed them of our almost total lack of knowledge about this 'last chance' serum."

The *Tribune* added that the Ottawa official also affirmed "no pressure whatsoever" had been put on any doctor who wanted to obtain authorization to use 714-X on patients:

Our role is not to encourage, or discourage, doctors on this. However, our responsibility is to say that a product has won no scientific recognition. And we must also inform physicians that, if there are repercussions, legal or otherwise, as a result of action by patients' families or by the Medical Corporation, Health and Welfare acquits itself of all responsibility in that regard. So the doctor acts at his own risk. That's why most of them have decided to back out.

Had the Canadian public had the opportunity to hear the almost incessant ringing of Gaston Naessens's Rock Forest doorbell and telephone or to listen to conversations on its line between the researcher and physicians calling in to inquire where they could get 714-X, and to report on favorable changes in patients already under treatment with it, Cléroux's statement that most doctors were "backing out" would seem most puzzling, to put it mildly.

Let us "listen in" on a typical exchange between Naessens and one of these doctors, who practices in a small town in the province of Ontario:

Naessens: Good evening, Doctor . . . I just received news that you've been treating Mr. B. with my 714-X.

Doctor: That's right!

Naessens: How's it going?

Doctor: Really nicely!

Naessens: Can you tell me about the case?

Doctor: Yes. He came to me with cancer of the left tonsil that had spread to his pharynx with extensions to the jawbone. He could no longer take nourishment and had to be fed through a tube into his stomach. After only fifteen days of injections with 714-X, he's begun eating normally again—ravenously—he's hungry all the time. He's almost off painkilling narcotics. And there are lumpy masses on his body that have become inflamed in a reaction suggesting that something in them is dying. The man is so happy! He's got so much energy back, he's thinking of returning to work.

Naessens: I'm so pleased.

Doctor: I have another patient, a forty-year-old woman with cancer in both breasts. Ottawa has approved treatment, which she wants to take right here. Can you send me some more of the product?

Naessens: As soon as Ottawa authorizes me to do so. Do you inject it yourself?

Doctor: No. I haven't yet learned to do so. But I have a colleague who knows how. She says it's no big deal to learn the technique.

Naessens: That's right. It seems as if a lot of you can now move forward with me, once you've realized 714-X isn't just a solution of "water and camphor."

Doctor (laughs heartily): Yeah, that's it!

Naessens: Let me ask you, when you spoke with the

Ottawa authorities, did they try to discourage you from using my product?

Doctor: Well, they did tell me what their position was—tried to put 714-X in a bad light—warned me I could be sued for using it. Despite all that, I just told them: "Look, I want it!" So they said they'd approved my request.

Naessens: Good. Because there have been several doctors who've told me they were counseled by Ottawa not to use my product.

Doctor: Sure. You could say the same for me. But I insisted on it.

Naessens: And you're not alone, Doctor. You know that, don't you? I now have a list of a dozen of your colleagues who've been sent 714-X and are using it right now.

Doctor: Wonderful! Can you give me your telephone number? So I can call you from my office in a few days and give you another report.

Naessens: (gives number).

Doctor: Can I get you at that same number after supper?

Naessens: Yes.

Doctor: Okay, thank you. I'll be calling you in a few days.

Naessens: Thank you, Doctor. Good night.

While Naessens's morale was now high, it had never been low, not even during the trial. As he would later tell a journalist interviewing the "human being" rather than the "scientist": "I certainly am sure that I have always been guided by what you refer to as some kind of 'higher force.' It's nothing extraordinary, but I believe in God, and in what I'm doing. Had I not that gift of faith, I don't know whether I would have made it through so many of life's trials without going mad. I am not at all ashamed to admit that I ask help from the Divine. I know that justice awaits, if not here on earth, then on a higher plane. That is why I'm glad to have entered a fight to demonstrate the worth of my discoveries over the last forty years."

On the matter of what "allies" he had to help him win acceptance for his treatment in the medical field, he said: "Look, the corporation has tried to stick a label on me. But the public is no dupe, so there'll be winds of change blowing. If, as Dr. Fabre said in court, all doctors could act out of 'soul conscience,' you'd see really radical changes in the health field!"

And, on the subject of freedom in research: "Any researcher who is not free is no longer a researcher. If I were compelled to do work assigned by someone else, I'd lose all my creativity, my original thinking. On any research trail, there are many forks and new roads, which, if they are felt to lead somewhere, must be taken even if they travel away from the beaten track and one's original goals."

Chapter 14
The Quest for Truth

*My purpose is not to say that phenomena have been
proved, but to point out that however much proof was
or could have been provided, the phenomena are not
acknowledged as facts because they are so drastically at
variance with the prevalent interpretation of science . . .
this attitude is against the interests of true science and
is even contrary to elementary justice, for it becomes
impossible to correct a theory by experimental test as
long as theory decrees in advance what the outcome of
the test must be.*

Arthur Middleton Young,
The Reflexive Universe

Unlike a fairy tale, the story told here has no ending, far less
any "they lived happily ever after." An ideal *finis*, of course,
would portend that Gaston Naessens's new science becomes
widely known, that his microscope becomes duplicated to
allow researchers in hundreds of laboratories to view the
microbiological world it has revealed, and that his medicinal
products become everywhere available to patients who badly
need them. What on earth needs to happen for that to occur?

The question seems to reduce to the old paradox: "If
Mohammed won't go to the Mountain, must the Mountain
come to Mohammed?"

One scenario casts Gaston Naessens as a "scientific
prophet" who stubbornly refuses to make the long trek to
the scientific establishment's "Mount Olympus." As erected
by the research director for an American institute involved
in scientific investigation and public education—"St. Patrick,"
as we shall call him—it begins with the idea that, if Naessens

191

were only willing to *share* his work in the "normal" way—
that is, by publishing his findings in recognized scientific
journals—a "whole new world of biology would be opened up."

The problem with this dictum is that it seems to imply
unwillingness on St. Patrick's part to recognize that—whether
conventional science is aware of it or not—Naessens has *already* opened up that new world, and his use of the word
"normal" has a harsh ring to it.

In his now-classic book *The Structure of Scientific Revolutions* (Chicago: University of Chicago Press, 1962), Thomas
Kuhn referred to "normal" science, by which he meant the
"ruling scientific outlooks" dominating any given epoch. It
was Kuhn's central thesis that such outlooks could only be
swept away in favor of more novel ones through the creation
and ultimate acceptance of a new model, or worldview, which
he called a paradigm.* Unfortunately, the model was constrained to "wait in the wings"—for years and in some cases
even for centuries—until the ascendant dogmas of a "normal"
science finally ceded center stage to a "revolutionary" one.

For that to happen, Kuhn maintained, the "time" must
be "ripe." Other philosophers of science have more recently
subscribed to a view just as dreary. One of them, Gunther

---

*In his new book *Cross Currents* (Los Angeles: J.P. Tarcher, 1990),
Robert O. Becker, M.D., characterizes the medical paradigm that
has existed for forty years as "based on the chemical-mechanistic
concept of life. In this view, living things were chemical-mechanical
machines whose capabilities were constrained to those functions
permitted by this model; there was no place for any characteristics,
such as autonomy or self-healing, that did not fit this mold. This
view was reinforced until it became a dogma, the proponents of
which claimed to know everything there was to know about life.
This paradigm not only dominated our society but ruled the medical
profession as well, limiting both the methods that could be used
to bring about a cure and our perception of the ability of the human
body to heal itself."

Stent, writing about the problem of a scientist's reporting something entirely novel, such as Naessens's *Nu* biology, suggests that such data often falls into a category of being too premature.* In Stent's somewhat ponderous definition: "A discovery is premature if its implications cannot be connected by series of simple logical steps to *canonical*, or generally accepted, knowledge [my emphasis]." Canonical? Does not the theological overtone of that word suggest—as Beverly Rubik so concisely put it—that science has "taken on the behavior of its early oppressor: the church"?

In presenting examples of what he considers to be important premature discoveries, Stent brings up one that is particularly relevant to the case of Gaston Naessens. In 1869, he writes, Friedrich Miescher discovered DNA in the cell nucleus, and speculation began that it might have some function in heredity. But the idea was only finally accepted in 1952, or seventy-five years later, even though Oswald Avery had, in fact, made the discovery that DNA was responsible for heredity in 1944.

One of Naessens's most awe-inspiring findings, made circa 1969, a century after Miescher's, and proved in his experiments with rabbits, is that the somatid, as a DNA precursor, plays a hitherto unknown role in heredity. Is this finding to be considered as "premature" as Miescher's and, if so, will it take another seventy-five years to confirm?

The "prematurity" factor brought out in Stent's article more than pessimistically implies that ideas presented "before their time" are, because too "strange," simply not *welcome* to science, just as new strains of apples, harvested and

*Gunther Stent (University of California at Berkeley) "Prematurity and Uniqueness in Scientific Discovery," *Scientific American*, December 1972. I am beholden to Brendan O'Regan, vice president for research, Institute of Noetic Sciences (Sausalito, California), for drawing my attention to Stent's article.

marketed in summer, might appear suspect to purchasers used to buying apples in the fall.

With respect to Naessens's somatoscope, St. Patrick asks: "What is preventing it from being shared?" The question implies that, once again, it is Naessens's very unwillingness to let his instrument out of his laboratory or, better still, get it manufactured in series, that has also blocked wider recognition of his findings.

Not a little incomprehensibly, St. Patrick adds, "Would Galileo have ever gotten very far if there were only *one* telescope in the world?" Is this meant to suggest that the Italian astronomer, after being put on his knees by the papacy and forced to recant his discoveries, was supposed to have become a telescope manufacturer?

We have seen in the pages of this book that, with regard to Naessens's microscope, letters from microscopic experts in two German optical companies have lauded it as the most advanced of its kind in the world. How is it that their executives have taken no *initiative* to assist Naessens in its development and distribution?

Finally, with respect to dissemination of information through "normal" channels, we may point out that, since American President Nixon "declared war" on cancer in 1971, "information" diffused by the cancer establishment has filled thousands upon thousands of pages in monographs and journals. By 1988, expenditure for research and treatment of the disease had cost over one trillion dollars! All of this money, effort, and time was mostly spent on the basis of the existing cancer paradigm, the "normal" idea, that, as brought out by Dr. Fabre in Naessens's trial, cancer cells can only, and therefore must, be destroyed by a cytotoxic — cell-killing — method.

On the other hand, Naessens's "revolutionary" outlook, espoused for over forty years, has run counter to that dominant philosophy. That "Mohammed" has cured a great many people of cancer seems to make not the slightest difference to the denizens of "Mount Olympus." When will the time be "ripe" for a paradigm shift in cancerology?

A completely different scenario puts the onus of the dilemma not on the shoulders of Mohammed, but atop the peak of the immovable Mountain.

This scenario is painted both by Dr. Jan Merta de Velehrad, who, as we have seen, is one of the few researchers to have successfully repeated most of Naessens's work, and Dr. Walter Clifford, who came all the way from Colorado Springs, Colorado, to testify on Naessens's behalf at the second Wellington Hotel press conference held in the summer of 1989.

During a conversation in early January 1990, I asked Merta to comment on the Mohammed-Mountain paradox. "Let me first say," he began, "that Gaston Naessens is one of the most conscientious and dedicated individuals I have ever met, a man completely devoid of any 'ulterior' motive, or any motive other than an overall aspiration to bring new understanding into the biomedical arena and, in so doing, to serve mankind."

Pausing to give me a piercing look, Merta continued: "Before I go on, Chris, I want you to know that, because of the many corporate and scientific responsibilities I have been given over many years, dealing with hard facts and taking responsibility for my statements is, for me, a 'way of life.'

"Having hopefully made that clear, I shall now tell you that it is my utterly sad conclusion that Gaston Naessens has been *ostracized* by the medical and scientific communities *just because* he has come across revolutionary new data to lay bare brand new understanding and develop a highly innovative and novel technology. All of this, and more, cuts against the grain of established dogma, of vested interests of all kinds, interests that control many, if not all, facets of our lives."

This statement seemed to me to reflect a concealed facet of Kuhn's "paradigm-shift" conundrum and Stent's "prematurity factor," the facet of *vested interest* lying at the heart of each of them, one that both professors leave out of their theses, perhaps because they considered it too ungenteel for academic discourse.

Merta was far more "hard-boiled." "This ostracism," he went on, "has *nothing* to do with Gaston's education and competence, or the lack of them. His fate is the fate of anyone who would dare to follow the same path he has walked in order to achieve the same results. I do not doubt for one second that, even should he win a Nobel prize, or equivalent honor, he would nevertheless be treated with silence and contempt.

"For it is not just the man, Gaston, but his ideas, his *Nu* biology, that the orthodox cannot stomach. The very intensity of the resistance to these ideas on many fronts suggests, in itself, that one fine day they will break through, in all their importance, to provide full employment for scientific, and other, workers in years to come." A "fine day." To dawn after a paradigm shift?

Merta also took a line on Naessens's microscope that went in a completely different direction from the one taken in St. Patrick's allusion to Gaston's not being willing to "share" it. "Over the years," he said, "I have seen many novel innovations, including some unusual microscopes. As one who has a command of optical technology, I can unequivocally say that, to my knowledge, there nowhere exists a microscope capable of matching the qualities of the one developed by Gaston Naessens. There is no 'mystery' to that instrument. It is easy to re-create. Given some time, and the proper equipment, I know I could do so myself.

"It is so easy to reproduce that it could well be 'taken over'—stolen—by any person or group who then could, and probably would, call it 'their own.' Even if that were done,

I have a strong suspicion that, given the present-day 'workings' of science, its recreation will not take place if only because, if it is manufactured in series and more widely distributed, it will first and foremost reveal a mass of erroneous scientific beliefs, not to say lies, and destroy existing scientific prejudices.

"The same vehemence with which the scientific and medical establishment keeps trying—as it has tried for forty years—to destroy Naessens's work and reputation will, I am afraid, be used to destroy his microscope."

"What is the main reason for the resistance to Naessens's discoveries?" I asked.

"It is an unfortunate fact that medicine is not motivated to search for truth," replied Merta. "The forces behind it are those that promote, not *healing and succor*, but *money and profit*. Good health, after all, is bad for 'business.' Because Gaston Naessens has offered, and offers, good health for a tiny fraction of the cost which, these days, people are forced to pay for a bad one, he is simply not wanted, together with what he has discovered.

"As a single individual, Gaston Naessens has achieved more than dozens of institutes full of Ph.D.s that have been supported, year after year, by millions and millions of dollars. My own experience as an inventor has taught me, to my rue, that most people have an *inborn* resistance to anything new, especially to anything they themselves have not invented or conceived. And many of them can only see what they want to see, just as if they were pickpockets trying to find a pocket on the diaphanous dress of an angel.

"You, yourself, wrote in your article in the *New Age Journal* what Walter Clifford, a veteran bacteriological scientist, had to say at a press conference held on behalf of Naessens last summer, which we both attended. I remember his words, which rang in my ears: 'My colleagues and I have found to our dismay that if you don't *toe the company line*, medi-

cal pundits don't even want to know what you've discovered,
whatever it might be.'"*

As Merta repeated these words, I berated myself for not
having followed up on an earlier decision to call Walter "Jess"
Clifford and ask him if he could expand on them. Reached
in his Colorado Springs home, he promised he would put a
short essay into the mail within twenty-four hours. The following passages from it show that Jan Merta was not the only
"artist" painting a darker scenario on the future of Naessens's
research.

"In most worthy endeavors," the essay begins, "there are
a few gentle giants who mold the age they live in. Gaston
Naessens is such a man. Generally, these master builders are
openly ridiculed by those styling themselves as 'learned.' I
refer to them as pygmies, not the little men of short bodily
stature, but pygmies in the *moral* sense of the word." Keepers
of the jail of the paradigm?

None of Naessens's detractors, people who do not
even seek to understand that there is more to real science
than has ever crossed their imagination, have ever bothered
to work with him in his laboratory. I have, many times,
personally taken researchers of their stamp into my own
laboratory to demonstrate to them, from their own blood
samples, exactly some of the things Naessens has been

---

* As Merta spoke, I saw the wonder that was Royal Raymond Rife's
"Universal Microscope" in irreparable condition on the floor of a
San Diego garage where I had found it, and one of its "sister" instruments, disassembled on a laboratory bench outside Chicago by
"scientists" who never could figure out how to put it back together
again. (The only extant Rife microscope, taken to England before
World War II, by the "Physician Royal," Dr. Gonin, was, after an
arduous search to find it, finally discovered by Jan Merta in the Well-
come Museum in London.) With one or two exceptions, a vast archive of photos taken with the "Universal Microscope" have also,
for whatever reason, disappeared off the face of the earth.

reporting for years. They viewed these things in my own microscope, things they've never seen before. Do you think that made any difference? As outrageous as it may seem, most of them unblinkingly told me that, because what they had seen was not approved by any professional society, or governmental agency, they simply *would not believe it.* Believe their own eyes, that is!

If these researchers, and I'm referring to dozens of them, were only dealing with abstractions, one might not necessarily be so profoundly shocked. But all of them, in one way or another, are supposedly responsible for *human life.* You may ask, "How can they be so callous?" The answer is connected to the *fear* they have of those who rule the medical and scientific fiefdoms of which they are only the vassals, fear that the power wielded by government agencies, drug companies, or research foundations will cut off their little funding grants and put an end to their "careers," if they step out of line. So they kowtow to authority and limit themselves to discovering exactly what their liege lords want them to discover, as thousands of worthless published research papers indubitably prove.

Like Merta, Clifford was unveiling a brand new facet of the "paradigm" and "prematurity" problems left unmentioned by Kuhn and Stent.

Any project aimed at replicating and substantiating Gaston Naessens's work will never fit into the program of grant applications of any major funding organization that I know of. The very simplicity of the task mitigates against this. Naessens's investigations require no "megabuck" irradiation machines, scanners, or other costly and complex equipment. And his findings will certainly not sell billions of dollars worth of toxic drugs.

Echoing Jan Merta, Walter Clifford next pointed to the ease of replicating all of Naessens's techniques and findings:

His work can be learned with no great difficulty by any reasonably skilled technician. His products can be made in laboratories containing the most modest facilities, and be administered by virtually any family physician. As a professional in the field, I can further say that the microbiology involved in them can be duplicated by any researcher willing to accept a body of new knowledge of vast importance that never has been taught in a university or a medical school.

This whole body of knowledge had, in the courtroom, been dismissed by Dr. Lorenzo Haché as "marginal."

Ending his essay on a personal note, Clifford concluded:

The peculiar microbiology and life cycles found in Naessens's research have been an inspiration to me. It has been my good fortune, and privilege, to have worked in parallel with some of his work. From my own independent investigations, which predate my first acquaintance with him, I know the truth and value of the principles he espouses. Those colleagues with whom I have shared this work, men and women willing to put prejudices and preconceptions aside in order to open-mindedly evaluate it, have found it to be as great a revelation as have I.

In other words, those who do not consider the work "premature."

"There is some hope that Naessens's magnificently original work will spread out, but I can say, Chris, that winning the minds and hearts of professional scientists and medical researchers, not to speak of firing their determination to go against the 'crowd,' will be, by far, not as simple as winning a legal battle in a courtroom." With those words, Clifford provided one answer to the question asked at the opening of this chapter. And he bolstered my idea that only people tugging on a second rope might, in the end, drag Naessens's work forward: "I believe you are right when you told me over the telephone that it may be only 'old-fashioned people power' that will have to win the day for Naessens, with whom I am honored to stand side by side at any time."

Can "people power" break the scientific paradigm? The idea would shock the temple of science, whose priests have never welcomed the idea that mere people have any say in the politics determining the direction of their pursuits, or the writing of their "canon."

That the paradigm will one day be broken Jan Merta de Velehrad has no doubt. "The time will surely come," he told me, "perhaps in the next century, when science will realize it has proceeded in many wrong directions, even up 'blind alleys.' Only at that time will Gaston Naessens's work, like the work of other pioneers in other fields of endeavor, be recognized as having offered a 'way out.' But, until that time comes, most people will neither want, nor dare, to 'see,' to 'hear,' to 'speak out,' or to 'step forward.' Such giants as Royal Raymond Rife, Wilhelm Reich, and others, along with a few supporters, had the courage to do so, and the price they paid was a heavy one, the price of *martyrdom*."*

Jan Merta shot me another piercing look. "I want you to know, Chris," he said solemnly, "that, with regard to what I have told you, I have not been exaggerating. It has been my central aim in life to search for *valid information*, that is, for truth, no matter how unacceptable or premature it may be considered by the 'orthodox,' no matter how upsetting to the 'reigning paradigm.' For man's judgment is only as good as the information available to support it."

---

*Reich died in a Federal penitentiary, and two of Rife's loyal assistants were sentenced to terms of imprisonment.

Part Four
The Battle Continues

Chapter 15
Gladiators in a New Arena

*At the heart of science lies discovery which involves
a change in worldview. Discovery, in science or the arts,
is possible only in societies which accord their citizens
the freedom to pursue the truth where it may lead and
which therefore have respect for different paths to the truth.*
John Polanyi, Canadian Nobel Laureate (Chemistry),
from his commencement address at McGill University,
Montréal, June 1990

How does information, valid as it might be, become widely
accessible when it is cleverly concealed or censored? It is
about that question that Jan Merta had nagging doubts. As
1990 wore its way from winter into spring, and then into summer, the search for truth in Québec, with respect to Gaston
Naessens's revolutionary discoveries as revealed at the trial,
seemed hardly being pursued by those best equipped to do
so, namely, the media monopolies that mold public opinion.

That Naessens's victory in the judicial arena was epic
in proportions is made indubitably clear by a letter written
to me shortly after the trial by Peter Weldon, Esq., a senior
legal counselor in Sherbrooke, who had taken time off from
his professional duties to be present during testimony of various witnesses, and summing up by counsel. "In retrospect,"
Weldon wrote on the stationery of his law firm, "I can say
without hesitation that the Naessens trial, *one of the most
important in legal and social terms to have taken place in
recent Canadian history,* represents a great step forward in
public recognition and vindication of unorthodox pioneers
in the vital field of alternative medicine."

Given that unequivocal statement about Naessens's

court triumph, it is more than amazing that no Québécois, or, for that matter, Canadian, journalist writing for a leading newspaper or periodical has yet seen fit to write an article echoing Weldon's pronouncement on the precedent-setting trial. Nor has any science writer of note bothered to investigate and report on the substance of Naessens's discoveries so that people everywhere might understand their vast scope. Had they been written, such articles might, at the very least, have evoked pride in a provincial populace that it was one of their fellow citizens, working in a tiny private laboratory, who had opened a whole new scientific frontier and who had been recognized for his achievements with a verdict of "Not Guilty."

The final section of this book attempts to get to the bottom of this dilemma, and to report on what has transpired during the first half of the year 1990. What is the nature of the dilemma of great concern to society at the end of this millennium? One answer concerns the lack of any real respect for a verdict passed by that society's system of justice on the part of that same society's overlords in the medical field.

It is as if medical "dictatorship," a hegemony in its own right, stands, as we shall see, outside newly developing social "norms," and aloof from a general social wisdom that inherently senses a "con game" promulgated by health practitioners in the ascendancy. The most blatant indication of this, in the wake of Naessens's jurisprudential triumph, was a counterattack against what his trial had revealed, mounted by three minions of the Québec Medical Corporation—cancer men all—to destroy the significance of that courtroom milestone, as so clearly underscored by Peter Weldon.

This counterattack came in the form of a formal press conference, televised throughout the province of Québec on prime time, from an auditorium in Montréal's Nôtre Dame Hospital, where it was chaired by a leading young cancer specialist, Dr. Jacques Jolivet.

Five weeks prior to the press conference itself, Jolivet

had been invited by popular Québec television host Pierre Nadeau to appear on his interview program, "Sept Jours de Tele-Metropole." The broadcast showed Jolivet talking with Naessens and committing himself to set up a clinical verification of the effectiveness of 714-X in the fight against cancer. As one of Naessens's loyal supporters said to me: "At last one could hope that the 'Naessens Affair' would be settled and brought to its denouement, one way or the other."

It was not until 21 February that Jolivet finally trekked to Rock Forest, where he spent nearly a whole day talking with Naessens and his wife, with whom he enjoyed a home-cooked lunch prepared by Françoise. In the laboratory, where he inexplicably showed not the slightest interest in viewing samples of healthy or unhealthy blood at Naessens's microscope, the physician had the opportunity to look over, and to examine closely, more than two dozen medical dossiers of patients who had benefited from 714-X treatment, including one "open-and-shut" case from Dr. Michel Fabre in France on a man who had completely recovered from lung cancer, a case on which Fabre had earlier provided sworn testimony at the trial.

But, no matter how impressive or convincing all these summaries might have seemed to other observers, oncologist Jolivet insisted to Naessens that every one of them had certain "flaws," or "weaknesses," as far as their being able to fulfill international standards established by cancerologists for reporting cancer "cures."

Still, Jolivet seemed far from being wholly negative. It appeared that he was sufficiently impressed to be able affably to inform Naessens that he would be glad to work on the dossiers and correct various deficiencies in them so as to bring them "up to standard." Naessens was as much overjoyed by Jolivet's offer as by the courteous manner of its presentation. When the two men said their good-byes, the independent researcher was heartwarmingly convinced that he had finally gained a true ally within the ranks of orthodox cancer specialists.

Imagine Naessens's surprise, therefore, when Jolivet—whether under coercion by his medical superiors, or of his own free will—went back on his word. The very next day, he organized the cited conference at which he, together with two other cancer-specialist colleagues, sat at a raised podium to affirm to reporters from the printed and electronic media that cancer patients throughout Québec province should *expect no help whatsoever* from a product that he characterized not only as bogus but as potentially dangerous. It was as if the three-week-long trial, offering ample evidence to the contrary, had never been held.

One of the two other doctors taking part in the session was Gerald Baptist, who disparaged Naessens and all his research in a particularly snide and hostile manner. This physician had also earlier visited Naessens's laboratory, accompanied by a public television crew. In full view of the camera, which made an undeniable, if unwitting record of it, Baptist distorted the truth for thousands of TV viewers by reading lines from one dossier to the effect that treatment of the patient had been "ineffective." Unrevealed by Baptist was the fact that he was citing the lines wholly out of context, that is, they applied *not* to the case under discussion, but to the subject of a second, wholly different, file. Nor was Baptist at all ashamed to state, from the same podium, and in draconian tones, that 714-X should under no circumstances be used on any cancer patient, not even one terminally ill, because there was *no proof whatsoever* of its efficacity.

Even more monstrous was an apparent lie told by the panel's third cancer doctor, Jean Latreille, who falsely hinted that certain terminal cancer patients were dying in their hospitals, possibly due to the *highly toxic* effects of 714-X doses previously administered to them.

On the matters of efficacity and toxicity, court-attested evidence, diametrically opposed to the allegations of the two cancer doctors, seemed to make not the slightest difference to them.

Of the many journalists present, only one, Francine Ravinsky, had it in her to stand up to the medically inquisitorial threesome. Tearing into Jolivet with five minutes of persistent and pointed questions, all of which he either dodged or refused to answer, she finally so exasperated the panel's chairman that he irritatedly, almost desperately, declared that the whole matter of Naessens and his 714-X was, in his eyes, as well as those of his colleagues and the Québec Medical College, a "case closed."

That, it seemed, was that. Québec medical power had once again imperially ruled from its throne. A cancer research "monarch" had spoken his final words to put the public, especially all cancer victims, once and for all on notice that they could give up all hope that 714-X could save them, or their friends and relatives.

Among hundreds, if not thousands, of Québécois citizens almost put into shock by Jolivet's harsh dictum was Maher Jahjah, the Egyptian-born editor and publisher of *Fusion*, a French-language magazine that specializes in questions of "frontier science." One of the few Québecers to take up the cudgels for Gaston Naessens in print, Jahjah, zeroing in on the central question of *concealment*, had brought out an article pointedly entitled "L'Affaire Naessens: Qui Câche Quoi?" (The Naessens Affair: Who's Hiding What?).

Jahjah was particularly incensed by the Medical Corporation's "mulish willfulness to preserve its *absolute hegemony* in the domain of health care" and by how strangely the facts of the Naessens case contrasted with the aseptic version of the story presented by establishment radio and television journalists. As he wrote: "It is sad indeed that the media seem to go along, if they do not openly side, with the corporation's outlook to give the public the impression that Naessens is only a charlatan touting a fraudulent product."

To counter the rank injustice of a one-sided presentation of the Naessens story, Jahjah teamed with François Bourbeau, director of a "Fusion" weekly television program with which the magazine of the same name is affiliated. Probing for an answer to the question "Who's Hiding What?," they decided to organize an "arm's-length debate" by inviting first Gaston Naessens, then Dr. Augustin Roy, for two separate hour-long interviews.

Prior to his on-screen talk with Naessens, Bourbeau made sure to do his homework. Together with his camera crew and a professional biochemist, he visited the Rock Forest laboratory to acquaint himself—as the cancer specialist had not—with the properties of the microscope about the optical qualities of which Jahjah was later to write, *"there was not a shadow of a doubt."*

As for Naessens's theories about the origin and development of degenerative disease, Jahjah characterized them as "extremely well articulated and certainly worthy of respectful attention by the whole scientific community." They reflected, he added, "the views of well-known American doctors, such as Carl Simonton and others, who had long held, just like Naessens, that while cancerous cells spontaneously appear regularly in all healthy persons, they are gotten rid of by a properly functioning immune system."

During the Rock Forest visit, reported Jahjah, Naessens demonstrated the very opposite of the "secretiveness" of which he had been accused by Dr. Roy. He had willingly given the "Fusion" TV team copious documentation* concerning his

---

*A great deal of this documentation had also been passed out to some dozen journalists at an earlier press conference to demonstrate that Roy's accusations that Naessens was prone to "hiding" data were false. Not a single line from it was alluded to, or printed, in the establishment press, broadcast over the air, or screened on TV.

research, he had carefully explained all of its technical aspects, and he had, as forthrightly as civilly, answered all of their many questions. Particularly impressive to the team was their opportunity to examine Naessens's "guest book," filled with the signatures and comments of visiting researchers from around the world.

In contrast to the open manner with which Naessens received the "Fusion" team, and his candidness during the TV interview itself, Augustin Roy, when he appeared in the studio for his own interview, seemed the epitome of secrecy. Although armed with a thick file on Naessens, which he claimed could supply "overwhelming evidence" of the biologist's scientific ineptitude and moral turpitude, he refused to turn over a single page on it, with the weak excuse that, beyond its being too "voluminous," it contained a few "surprises" for Naessens, "cats," as it were, that Roy did not want to let out of their "bag."

Jahjah had gone a long way toward answering the question "Who's Hiding What?" The answer clearly focused on the head of the Québec Medical Corporation and on public media overawed, if not intimidated, by the corporation. To pursue the matter further, the day following the televised press conference at Nôtre Dame Hospital, Jahjah put in a call to Dr. Jacques Jolivet. But, as he wrote in a subsequent article for *Fusion* magazine: "I not only found it impossible to get through to him, but was told that he was categorically refusing my own, or anyone else's, request to interview him on the subject of Naessens, or on any other."

Jahjah also revealed that Naessens had taken the trouble, during Jolivet's visit to his house and laboratory, to record their mutual conversation. "Is it that Jolivet," asked Jahjah in print, "aware that this recording was made, now doesn't wish to clarify the incoherence of his proposals in the light of his subsequent actions? We have listened to this recording, and we can confirm that Dr. Jolivet told Naessens that his medical dossiers were, in some ways, 'incomplete.' " It was not difficult to explain the "incompleteness," added Jahjah, the main reason for it being the fact that many patients, once brought back to health by Naessens's treatment, had refused to have anything more to do with doctors, or hospitals and their endless tests.

Confronting the issue of Jolivet's bad faith, Jahjah noted that, while Jolivet had told Naessens he would await, and examine, other dossiers necessary to decide the question, on the eve of the press conference Naessens had faxed him one file that exactly corresponded to the doctor's requirements, and Jolivet immediately rejected it out of hand.

Why, asked Jahjah, had Jolivet neither read all the documentation supplied him by Naessens nor circulated copies of it to his colleagues? How then could he and those same colleagues publicly assert that they had performed a *rigorous study* of 714-X that led to their "closing the book" on the Naessens case? If that was their definition of the word "rigorous," then it would seem there was plenty to worry about when it came to the same specialists administering so-called "scientifically proven" treatments.

"And," forcefully concluded the *Fusion* editor, "if it's exactly a lack of scientific rigor that Gaston Naessens is accused of, then why is it that even cancer specialists are beginning to admit that such treatments as chemotherapy are only expedients that *destroy*, far more than otherwise, the health of patients exposed to such treatments?"

In the conclusion to his second article in *Fusion* magazine, Maher Jahjah expressed the hope that it would be the health authorities at the national level, in the Canadian capital, Ottawa, rather than those of the province of Québec, who would finally unravel the question of the potential benefits of Gaston Naessens's 714-X. And, indeed, it seemed that the terrible finality of Dr. Jolivet's pronouncements happily extended no further than to the frontiers of his Francophone, or French-speaking, region of the country.

We have seen that, starting shortly after the trial was over, the ministry had begun to receive calls from physicians, the majority of them in Québec province itself, requesting 714-X for their patients—only those who were terminally ill to be sure, that is, for whom no orthodox cancer treatment any longer offered any hope. This action on their part took a great deal of "guts," as is the more understandable when one remembers the likes of a Gerald Baptist solemnly averring that Naessens's product was wholly ineffective, and ordaining that it should *never* be used.

Yet, even within the bureaucratic maze of the Canadian Health Ministry, there were countercurrents suggesting an ambivalent attitude. While it seemed publically to be approving Naessens's therapy under what is known as the "Emergency Drug Act," certain of its own "functionaries" seemed bent on putting as many road blocks as they could on the road traveled by the braver doctors seeking to help their patients.

One of many phone calls from such doctors overheard at Naessens's house suffices to illustrate this anomalous state of affairs:

Doctor: I found, Madame Naessens, that when I called Ottawa, a Dr. Belanger to whom I was referred was rather aggressive!

Françoise: Ah, you were talking to Belanger?

Doctor: Yes, it seems they've now decided what we doctors seeking to treat our patients with 714-X must now speak not to one, but to two, of their doctors before getting an authorization for it.

Françoise: That only creates one more aggravating delay. One requesting doctor was forced to wait for eight days before I got the authorization to send him the medicine.

Doctor: Well, they've stipulated that we have to talk with *two* of them. One calls and bothers me—that's the first time! Then another, Belanger, calls and bothers me a second time. Sometimes, if I can't take the call, I have to call back, and then they're not in. It's a time-consuming process . . .

Françoise: You said he was fairly aggressive?

Doctor: Yes! He told me 714-X was nothing but a placebo effect—even worse—it was pure chicanery!

Françoise: He said it was *chicanery*?

Doctor: *Quite openly!* Well, I was busy with a patient, so I wasn't in any mood to start an argument, I can tell you. And one certainly isn't in the mood for that if one knows it can end by his saying: "You won't get your authorization." So I ended up saying: "Look, I can't say whether it's a placebo effect or not. We'll talk about it in a year's time if my patient is still with us." And I added that he should be testing it in Ottawa on a whole group of patients, but, well, he was *very disagreeable*, but the other one, Dr. Klein, she was far more understanding. What more can I say? I'm not doing all this just for "kicks." I just have to put up with them.

Françoise: It would be nice if they'd show a little goodwill . . .

Doctor: Yes, it would. You know, what we're involved with here isn't anything that's going to offer a smooth ride . . . you know what I mean? We're up against some *real power*, so we can't be in any hurry! We've got to be patient . . .

Françoise: Well, it's forty years now that my husband has been patient!

Doctor: We have to continue to be patient. I'll send you the faxed authorization so you can send me the product. . . . So long!

Despite the ambivalence, by mid-May 1990, one section of the Health Ministry was showing signs of increasing interest in 714-X. Naessens received a call from one of its administrators politely asking him if he could prepare a formal protocol for treatment of a group of cancer victims—not just those terminally ill—under his supervision and with the co-operation of collaborating physicians.

Yet, once again, it seemed that one bureaucratic "hand" inside the ministry did not know what another "hand" was doing. When Naessens reported this news to a group of journalists, they called the public relations section of the ministry, only to be informed that that office knew of no such invitation to present the protocol. Pressing for further information, the journalists were sent by fax only the obsolete communiqué its Québec regional headquarters had issued in January to the effect that 714-X was worthless. As usual, the press seized on the communiqué rather than on what Naessens had reported to it.

To prepare a protocol over one hundred pages in length is a long and a time-consuming task, especially for a man and his wife, working all alone, with neither secretarial or other logistic help. Just to find time available for this task was, by mid-June, becoming increasingly difficult, due to the exigencies of getting out 714-X—plus forty pages of information about it and instructions for its use—to the doctors, now numbering over fifty, who were requesting it.

Adding to Naessens's difficulties was the fact that, as Maher Jahjah had pointed out, the researcher had had a hard time obtaining documented attestations, signed by doctors of medicine, or hospital authorities, that would *confirm* the positive results 714-X was having on cancer cases.

Nevertheless, little by little, and after hundreds of hours of work, Naessens was able to gather together a thick file of medical dossiers bound in a volume that, one by one, had become available to him.

Some of these cases, added to those reported earlier in this book, go back to the pretrial time, when Naessens was himself administering the treatment. Let us look at six of the most interesting ones:

(1) As early as 1977, a fifty-two-year-old man was diag-

nosed with an adenocarcinoma (cancer of the lymphatic ganglia) in his prostate. Admitted to the hospital on 6 December, he underwent an exploratory operation, following which the hospital's "cancer committee" recommended the excision of the prostate itself plus all cancerous tissue in its immediate surroundings. This stern advice was adamantly refused by the patient, who also, and just as resolutely, turned down any other "aggressive" form of treatment.

Instead, the patient opted for 714-X treatment, which, beginning on 15 December, went through three series of twenty-one daily injections. In 1989, while in the hospital for reasons unconnected with his prostate cancer, the man was put through several tests, none of which could reveal a trace of cancer in his body.

(2) On 4 July 1980, a forty-five-year-old man was diagnosed with an epithelioma of the left vocal chord, a cancer that had metastasized to other parts of his body. The afflicted tissue did not disappear even after 1,000 rads of radiation, administered as part of a 6,000 rad dose, the maximum allowable because any higher dose would be likely to kill the patient.

On 15 July, the patient, who by that time had received a total of 1,500 rads, refused more such treatment, which was causing him great discomfort. Warned by doctors about the grave consequences that might ensue from his decision, he stuck to his guns. Starting on 16 September, he received three consecutive series of twenty-one injections of 714-X. In June 1990, or nearly ten years later, the same patient was in perfect health, and there had been no recrudescence of his illness.

(3) In December 1982, a fifty-nine-year-old woman was diagnosed with a malignant nodular lymphoma. Tests, including a chest X ray, a scan, and a biopsy, revealed that cancer had spread to the left and right lobes of her liver and, even more ominously, to her bone marrow. The hospital's "cancer committee" could do no more than to give the woman,

in a *terminal* condition, the standard advice: "Begin chemo-therapy forthwith!"

When this woman, who was well-informed about the shortcomings of such treatment, also adamantly refused to take it, she was started on 714-X treatment on 12 January 1983 under the supervision of her physician. Though she received only a single twenty-one-day treatment, this cancer patient, who was dying more than seven years earlier, was, in mid-1990, in good health with no reappearance of cancer.

(4) In December 1989, a twenty-three-year-old man was diagnosed with lymph ganglia cancer (multiple adenopathy) in the area above his collarbones on both sides of his body as well as in the pelvic region behind the right renal vein. His doctor accepted the patient's request to be treated with 714-X under the "Emergency Drug Act" as allowed by the health authorities in Ottawa. After four series of injections of 714-X, various tests performed on 16 March 1990 indicated that he had no more signs of cancer in his body. By June, the patient, facing death six months before, had gone back to work and was feeling in tip-top shape.

By early July, 1990, other doctors having the courage to treat cancer patients under the "Emergency Drug Act" were also reporting what to many of them seemed "unbelievable" changes for the better in the terminally ill, changes they had never seen in their years-long practices.

(5) One of these reports concerned a fifty-four-year-old woman who had come down with a case of colon cancer with metastases to her liver and lungs. Told she was no longer treatable with orthodox methods and that she could expect to live for no more than six months, cancer specialists sent her home to die.

On 21 February 1990, her doctor began 714-X treatment. By 3 March, she was able to be out of bed for most of the day, and her pain had significantly decreased. After three more series of injections, her doctor could report that she had "little or no pain" and that her heart, liver, and lungs were all "in good shape."

The patient went on with a fifth series of injections, following which her doctor reported "still more improvement." By October, the same patient had taken eight series of injections, at which point the doctor reported to the Naessenses that, clinically speaking, there was "continuing overall improvement of her condition and it was particularly important to note that her weight had stabilized at sixty kilograms." Since no side effects of the 714-X injections had been noted, he concluded, "we therefore wish to continue the injections."

(6) In November 1988, a fifty-seven-year-old woman was diagnosed with a cancerous kidney tumor. Her kidney was ablated. In October 1989, the cancer had spread to her lungs in the form of nodules, which began to grow in number and size. She was told that neither chemotherapy nor radiation could be of any benefit. Accordingly, the patient sought out 714-X treatment, which she began receiving on 21 February 1990. At first, this seemed ineffective, since, by 30 April, the number of nodules was still increasing and they were becoming larger. But, by 25 July, no new nodules were appearing, and the diameters of some on the existing ones were decreasing. In early September, all traces of the cancerous nodules had completely disappeared, and the patient was considered free of disease.

Some of the 714-X treatments have been "outside the system." A pair of moving letters from a patient and her doctor who obtained the product not through Ottawa, but clandestinely, were added to many reposing in Naessens's files. Wrote Dr. B: "I'd like very much to thank 714-X for its effective help to my patient. To our mutual satisfaction, I'm pleased to find out that that course of treatment, as developed by yourself, is presently making a very good clinical effect. One which will continue in the future, I hope. My sincerest gratitude and congratulations."

As for the patient, she herself wrote:

I wish to thank Monsieur Naessens for having developed the 714-X formula. Ever since I have been treated with it, I feel an increasing sense of well-being. The medical faculties believe that chemotherapy will help patients. But, talking from my experience, I can say that not only did it not help me, but made me feel much worse. I became very weak, was rapidly losing my vision and was shaking most of the time. My doctor has told me he has never before seen such a case as mine in which cancer was arrested after having become so widespread. God bless Monsieur Naessens!

While obviously no one would, or could, expect that all terminal patients would make as sensational, not to say incredible, recoveries as those just listed, even the ones who, following 714-X treatment, succumbed to cancer were in most cases offered great palliative benefits, which eased the final weeks of their lives.

Typical was the case of a fifty-seven-year-old man with cancer of the stomach and metastases to the liver who had stopped taking food and was unable to walk. After the first twenty-one-day series of 714-X injections, he was able to eat again and could take walks lasting up to fifteen minutes. Though, after four more series of injections, this patient finally died, during his last weeks of life he was entirely free of pain and was able to converse lucidly with his family. His life had been peacefully protracted for six months, after cancer specialists had given him no more than three weeks to live.

A second patient in this category was a fifty-nine-year-old woman with rectal cancer plus metastases. After an operation, she was so weak that her doctor, who did not expect her to live out the month, consented to administer 714-X as a "humanitarian" gesture to please the patient and her family, although he strongly doubted it would exert anything more than the "placebo effect," as the Health Ministry's Dr. Belanger had characterized it.

After a single twenty-one-day treatment, the doctor was able to report that his patient had ceased vomiting on a daily basis and had an increased appetite. A racking cough had all but disappeared. The patient was so encouraged by her improvement that she requested a second series of shots. This case is included here if only to illustrate how 714-X was able to improve the general condition of a mortally ill patient and to stress, once again, that if the same product is used in the *early* stages of cancer, before body-destroying orthodox treatments are used, the chances of its ridding the body of that disease are immeasurably enhanced.

That being the case, it seems highly ironic that the Canadian federal health authorities were, in 1990, allowing the 714-X treatment only for *terminal* patients and, in so doing, supporting the claim of the cancer establishment that orthodox treatments alone should be used to save the lives of cancer victims.

While dealing with all the problems linked to his fight to win a battle in the arena of "medical politics," Naessens was also facing a return to the legal arena. Even his magnificent victory in the 1989 court battle had not taken him off the juridical "meat hook" to which he seemed all but permanently impaled by the Medical Corporation. Throughout the first half of 1990, a second trial loomed over Naessens like a dark cloud. In the new proceedings, the Medical Corporation was to bring sixty-four charges—or counts—for "illegal practice of medicine," most of the infractions dating to 1984.

If set at a minimum of $5,000 per count, monetary fines could potentially amount to a whopping $380,000 and, if they were actually imposed, Naessens would have to find the money to pay them or go to jail.

As the time of Naessens's second trial approached, his defense lawyer, Conrad Chapdelaine, called him and his wife to a long conference at which he told them that, this time, he would mount a full-scale *offensive* with respect to the Medical College and its representatives and members, and "take the gloves off."

To implement this decision, he sent subpoenas not only to Dr. Augustin Roy, the Medical College's president, but to Drs. Jolivet, Baptist, and Latreille, who had organized the press conference. The lawyer's idea was to inveigle, or force, them to repeat *under oath* the detrimentally dishonest statements they had publicly made about Naessens and his work, and thus possibly subject them to countersuit for libel and/or whatever else might be applicable.

When the Naessenses informed me of Chapdelaine's new gambit, I wrote in my diary: "If victory in the first trial might be seen as a passive one, akin to the rescue of the bulk of the British army at Dunkirk at the start of World War II, Chapdelaine's intended strategy this time seems the legal analogue of the Normandy invasion that first ruptured the walls of 'Fortress Europe.'"

But the "invasion" was never to take place, the main reason being that the "enemy," to continue the military metaphor, began to retreat from its solidly entrenched positions before it could be launched. The "invaders," Naessens and his lawyer, were thus unable to demonstrate publicly their fighting ability.

And their adversaries, even in retreat, could be seen still to have the "upper hand." To understand why this was at all possible, one should know that to get medical doctors to appear in court, something which most of them wish, at all costs, to avoid, is not as easy as simply issuing mandates for that appearance. In fact, all the subpoenaed doctors were able to present reasons why they could not show up on the day appointed, or why their appearances would have to be postponed, perhaps interminably. In one sense, such an option might seem to put doctors as a class "above the law," but even if that point were debatable, it was obvious that this kind of "stalling game" could be protractedly played out to hold matters in abeyance for months, and to keep Naessens under cruel pressure.

On the other hand, a sure sign that the Medical College was feeling pressure of its *own* , due to Chapdelaine's aggressive action, was its countering with a "plea-bargaining" offer. As initially tendered, it proposed to drop half the charges if Naessens would plead guilty to the other half.

Over the telephone, Chapdelaine, digging in, categorically refused the offer and countered that he expected something much, much better or, otherwise, it would be "all systems go" for his original "battle plan." That the Medical College had serious qualms about entering any such foray became much clearer when, at six o'clock the same evening, in a further retreat, it offered to accept a guilty plea on only twelve charges, providing they included some of the most serious ones.

Continuing to "hang tough," Chapdelaine replied, "No deal!" The minimum he would accept was a guilty plea on ten charges, all of them applying to a single patient, Madame Langlais, and representing only the ten successive visits she had made to receive treatment from Naessens. And he added that, given the fact that it had been clearly proven in court that Langlais was a "goner" *before* those treatments were administered as a "last chance," he would accept only a minimal fine of $500 for each count, or a grant total of $5,000.

It was this demand to which the Medical College's lawyer, Roland Veilleux, finally acceded the following morning when he arrived at the Sherbrooke Palais de Justice. The Medical College had been put to flight. And an important reason

might well have been the fact that most of the cancer victims, some sixteen in all, implicated in the fifty-four charges
dropped by the college, had had the decency and the courage
to sign a document attesting to their being unwilling to testify that Naessens had treated them. They were courageous
in that such refusal, if they held to it, could expose them to
charges of "contempt of court" and, consequently, a term in jail.

The professional Medical Corporation's *revirement,* as
the French word has it, its "swing-around," or, in nautical
terms, its tack—even its *jibe*—was, in Chapdelaine's eyes,
a sign of acquiescence that Naessens simply could not refuse.
He further judged that the change of course, on the college's
part, was an important sign that things "were evolving in his
client's favor." As a veteran lawyer, he knew that, in any legal case of this type, it was best to follow the "least arduous
road." As he told the Naessenses: "When one has been able
to exact so large a tribute, there's no use asking for the moon!"

To allay any doubt on that score that the Naessenses
might still have, their lawyer continued in the same vein as
they and I sat with him at lunch in "Da Tony," one of Sherbrooke's most agreeable Italian restaurants, nearby the courthouse. While enjoying his poached salmon, Chapdelaine went
on to say that a long second trial, which would ensue if the
final plea bargain were not accepted, might well make "mar-
tyrs" of Madame Langlais and her husband and her relatives
in the eyes of the press and the public.

Over coffee, the attorney went further. "Even the college's official representative, present in court this morning,
seems highly relieved about the bargain we have made. To
me, that is one more sure indication that the doctors have
little appetite for a tough scrap."

"But, wouldn't *that* have been something?" Françoise
Naessens said a little dreamily.

"Sure," smiled Chapdelaine wolfishly, "and you know I
normally don't shrink from a legal fight! But on occasion, as

in this case, I know when to quit if circumstances dictate!"

After the judge passed formal sentence in the afternoon, at a subsequent short press conference, Chapdelaine made it perfectly clear that *despite* Naessens's acceptance of guilt on ten out of sixty-four charges, he had won what amounted to a "technical knockout," and that *despite* the charges that had been brought against him by provincial medical authorities, he had gained serious recognition at the Federal level. And to add weight to this assertion, it was revealed that, by 14 June, at least thirty-five doctors had been using 714-X on patients with the ministry's quasi-blessing.

While the accent of most press reports was placed not on the "giant step" backward taken by the Medical Corporation, but only on the fact that Naessens had pleaded guilty, a serious newspaper for French-speaking intellectuals, Montréal's *Le Devoir* (Duty) saw fit to include in its report that, as Chapdelaine had noted, "a certain form" of collaboration was beginning to be erected between Health Ministry specialists, various doctors, and his client, Naessens.

Chapter 16
Breakout From Québec

The history of many innovations, both in medicine and in other areas of endeavor, indicate that the innovators are often erratic, unsystematic, and difficult to deal with. The quality controllers often regard the work as of poor quality and not worth publishing or noting. . . . The only problem is that the quality controllers, while exquisite in their crossing of t's and dotting of i's, rarely discover anything that matters. The improvement of research quality over the past years is not gain if it has occurred at the expense of innovation.

David F. Horrobin, D.Phil., "The Philosophical Basis of Peer Review and the Suppression of Innovation," *Journal of the American Medical Association,* 9 March 1990

As well done as they were, the *Fusion* articles, both of them, seemed to skirt, or miss, the overridingly most important of Naessens's discoveries, the "jewel in their crown": the discovery of the somatid, along with its extraordinary properties and fascinating implications for biological and medical science.

The first medical recognition of the importance of that tiniest of microbiological entities came to me in a letter from the United States written by Karl Maret, M.D., trained in the "anthroposophic" tradition of Austrian scientist and clairvoyant Rudolph Steiner. Maret, who is also an engineer, heads the Metanoia Group in San Diego, California, which investigates areas indicated by Steiner as being of great interest for "future science."

Among Steiner's clairvoyant feats was his coming to conclusions, a few years before Gaston Naessens was born, about the true nature of cancer. Included with Maret's letter was a paper written by a German physician, which opens with the sentence: "As early as 1920, Rudolph Steiner described the malignant tumor as a disease of the organism *as a whole.*" This is exactly the philosophy adopted by Gaston Naessens — who had never heard of Steiner or his conclusion — over the course of his years-long independent research.

The German doctor next observed that, more than seventy years ago, Steiner tried to "direct attention away from the abnormal single cell environment, to extracellular space, and thereby to the permeable fluid continuum of that organism." And, amazingly enough, this is also what Naessens, who, using classical Greek humors to refer to "extracellular space," has tried to do all along, only to be vilified by a "cancer community" as ignorant of Steiner's reflections as if he had never existed, and as hostile to Naessens as if he were the foe, rather than the friend, of true medical science.

It seems odd, indeed, that Steiner's clairvoyant conclusions have not been heralded with avid interest by cancer specialists and that the truths he foresaw and proclaimed have not been recognized, especially since they have now been fully objectified by Naessens, who was born the same year Steiner died.

In his letter, Dr. Maret went on to ask a number of pertinent questions about the somatid, and other aspects of Naessens's research that not a single Québécois doctor or scientist seems to have mustered the curiosity to ask. This is hardly surprising. While the whole range of Steiner's scientific insights — what has been called a whole "Science of the Invisible" — create a revolutionary new vision in many disciplines, and thus require those studying them to think for themselves, orthodox medical teaching and training demands not personal and original inquiry, but largely rote learning. This is why brand new approaches are castigated, as they were in the Naessens's trial by Dr. Haché, as "marginal."

Let us set down some of Maret's questions and try to answer them in order to give some idea of what the medical community in Québec and elsewhere, and the popular science press, might, were they both "awake," also have been asking.

Question: How is it determined that somatids have electromagnetic negativity, and repulse one another?

Answer: They are easily seen to be repulsing one another at the microscope, just as if they were miniature equivalents of negatively charged billiard balls, which, on the green baize of a pool table surface, would never come in contact, or carom off one another, and thus make billiards an impossible game to play. Furthermore, they are attracted to the field of the positive pole of an ordinary magnet placed close to the blood sample on a slide.

Question: Is there information on the complete sixteen-stage life cycle of the somatid, published or written up in more detail (than provided in the book)?

Answer: While a "full-dress" scientific paper on this subject remains to be written, a videocassette film is readily available, over half an hour long, which shows most of the forms in the sixteen-stage cycle developing before one's eyes in the blood. The same film also includes still photographs of great interest to a comprehension of the functioning of the cycle.

Question: Have somatids, and other forms in the cycle, actually been seen in microscopes, but not been recognized?

Answer: Yes, most definitely. Over the years, many forms in the cycle have been observed by researchers in Europe and North America during a period stretching back to the 1920s, and beyond. A fascinating history of these observations remains to be written. A main difficulty, here, is that most of the observers were left puzzled by what they were seeing, either because they had found only some of the forms—usually the bacterial ones—but were unable to relate them to the rest of the cycle, and especially to the originating form, the somatid, which existing microscopes could not reveal. Or, because fellow bacteriologists simply dismissed the forms as "artifact," or dross, unwittingly or carelessly introduced into the milieu, and therefore not a natural part of it. This latter conclusion particularly applies to the sixteenth stage form, the empty *thallus*.

Question: How does Naessens's work relate to Dr. Virginia Livingston-Wheeler's—and others—on filterable bacteria?

Answer: Here Dr. Maret refers to a veteran physician, cancer researcher, and microbiologist who, before her recent death, operated a clinic in San Diego, California. Her conclusions about certain microbes she discovered and described seem to differ from those of Naessens mainly because she ascribes a cancer-*inducing* effect to them while Naessens insists that the sixteen-stage cycle is not a *cause*, but an *indicator* of disease, no different from a flashing light warning someone of incipient danger.*

The cancer-*causing* role of forms in the bloodstream derives from the old Pasteurian legacy that "germs" invade the body from without. Only a short time after Maret wrote to me, I received a paper, written by a Florida pathologist Dr. P. B. Macomber and printed in the British journal *Medical Hypotheses*, a leader in its field. The article, brought out in its first 1990 issue, summarizes years of research on anomalous microbes in the blood, but, once again for lack of knowledge of the somatid—originator of the whole process—it hews to the idea that microbes are *causes* for degenerative diseases, rather than their *heralds*.

Macomber's original interest in researching and writing his article came after his wife's death from cancer, which conventional therapy, in his words, "did not help at all . . . in fact

*See Appendix A for more on "filterable bacteria."

I think it *hastened her demise."* When he was introduced to
Livingston-Wheeler's research, he was flabbergasted. "I was,"
he continued in a letter to me, "upset, to say the least, that I
had never heard of any of the concepts about cancer that she
was developing even though, as a pathologist, I was reasonably familiar with most of the current research. No textbook
on oncology has even brushed on the subject."

No statement can better characterize the abyss that
yawns between orthodox philosophies on cancer and its treatment, and nearly a century of "new" knowledge, which, because it runs counter to those outlooks, has persistently been
ignored. Nevertheless, the receipt of the two communications, the one from a "Steiner" doctor, the other from a ranking pathologist suddenly brought face-to-face with a whole
"new world," seemed to promise that some people, somewhere, were at last beginning to throw a span across the abyss
of ignorance.

By the summer of 1990, as a result of limited dissemination of the English version of the Canadian-published book
abroad, more international support for Naessens's work was
shown by members of the international medical community
outside Canadian territory, support that more than matched
the goodwill and true interest evinced by the questions,
mostly of a theoretical nature, posed by Dr. Maret.

In Tijuana, capital of Mexico's Baja California state,
Mildred Nelson, a registered nurse and director of the Bio-
Med Center on Avenida General Ferreira, had read the Canadian edition of this book given her by Kim Lalancette, a
young Québecer who, like Bernard Baril and other young
AIDS victims, had recovered from his affliction after treatment
by Naessens's remedies. Leafing through its pages, Nelson,
a veteran battler for alternative cancer cures, grew increasingly
excited.

As far back as the 1930s, the Tijuana clinic director had
become chief assistant to Harry Hoxsey, a Texan oil million-

aire who had developed a formula made up of seven herbs,* plus potassium iodide, the earliest version of which his great-grandfather had first concocted in the mid–nineteenth century after watching a cancerous horse seek out special meadow plants, the ingestion of which led to recovery.

Used on hundreds of cancer victims, the Hoxsey formula's results were so promising that the American Medical Association (AMA) made its inventor a stingy offer to buy all rights to it. The offer, made in 1924, was flatly turned down by Hoxsey, who, as a result, became the object of a relentless AMA persecution, which, lasting for thirty-five years, was to lead to his repeatedly being charged with practicing medicine without a license and to his being sentenced to several jail terms.

Only Hoxsey's personal fortune, gained through his oil and gas ventures, allowed him to meet the legal costs of his extensive court battles and to continue to treat suffering cancer victims. In 1949, he carried his fight into enemy territory by suing the AMA.

The cake of his victory against America's most powerful medical authority was frosted when both the judge presiding at the trial and the AMA's own lawyer declared that there was no doubt that *Hoxsey's formula really did cure many cases of cancer.*

Yet, in spite of all this, and as incredible as it may seem,

---

*For another enthralling historical account of a Native American herbal remedy successfully used on cancer victims, and its suppression by the U.S. and Canadian medical authorities, see *ESSIAC: An Herbal Treatment of Cancer (A Special Report)*, by Tom Valentine, Associated Partners West, P.O. Box 3048, Iowa City, Iowa 52244. Unpublished is the testing of still one more herbal concoction obtained from the head-shrinking Jivaro Indians by the late Pino Turolla, an Italian explorer, and author of *Beyond the Andes* (New York: Harper & Row, 1980). Tested on cancer-infested mice in a Seattle, Washington, laboratory for over two years, it proved ninety-eight percent effective in stopping their cancers.

the AMA, with unbounded viciousness, kept hounding Hoxsey as a quack. Exhausted by his struggles, Hoxsey finally closed his clinics and moved his operation to Tijuana, where, since his death, Mildred Nelson has presided over it.*

Once she had finished reading my book about Naessens, Mildred Nelson immediately decided to send one of her five staff physicians to Rock Forest to learn Naessens's intra-lymphatic injection techniques for 714-X. In early June 1990, Al Espinosa, M.D., a handsome pure-blooded Olmec Indian in his midthirties, whose education from grade school all the way through medical school had been financed by Americans living in Guadalajara for whom Espinosa's mother worked as a housemaid, came to Naessens's laboratory. During the whole of an afternoon, he was shown the injection tech-niques, which were recorded on videocassette. He was fur-ther so well coached on the techniques in Montréal that, within two days, he had completely mastered them, and was skilled enough to be able to teach them to doctors and nurses in his *Tierra del Sol* homeland.

While it may seem strange that first evidence of intent to put 714-X treatment to practice had to come from an "al-ternative medicine" clinic, and from "south of the border," rather than from a leading hospital in the United States, it must be realized that, for American doctors to be able to use it, various "political" moves leading to legal "action" must be made for 714-X to somewhere acquire official status. Even if in Mexico it does not yet enjoy that official status, 714-X is nevertheless "tolerated" by state and medical authorities just because its nontoxicity and salubrious effects are recog-nized, a "tolerance" much to be desired in the fifty states of the American Union. But at least there is a clinic where

_____

*A prize-winning film, "Hoxsey," available on videocassette, was made by Ken Ausabel and can be obtained by writing to him at Box 1644, Santa Fe, New Mexico 87504.

Americans will be able to get the Naessens treatment while waiting for it to become available in their own country.

As Nelson was beginning 714-X treatment in Baja California, dozens of letters and telephone calls were pouring into the Naessens's house on Rue Fontaine from patients in the United States. They were advised that, since 714-X was legally exportable from Canada, it could be sent to them as soon as an American doctor mailed or faxed a written prescription for it. By mid-June, Françoise's log of prescriptions already sent was rapidly expanding. On 16 June, my own diary read: "Yesterday I traveled to a little Vermont post office just over the border to mail envelopes with instructions for the use of 714-X."

It is heartening to be able to write that Dr. Espinosa is not the only North American physician to have shown active interest in making 714-X available to patients. Lawrence Taylor, M.D., director of the U.S. Medical Research Foundation in San Diego, made his own trip to Rock Forest in early May 1990 to attend a reception celebrating the appearance of the Canadian edition, held for over two hundred Naessens partisans in Sherbrooke's new Delta Hotel. At the reception, Taylor rose to take the microphone and to congratulate Naessens graciously on his achievements on behalf of Taylor's American medical colleagues.

At the same reception, Naessens himself addressed the throng, and in moving words stated, not a little sardonically, that, myself excepted, "no scientifically trained observer had found any useful reason to monitor and relate all the details of my trial." My book, he added, "went far beyond the sterile polemics broached by persons who have no eyes to see, even less to understand, new approaches being advocated by various scientists in the domain of fundamental biological research." The book was "a trumpet blaring to awaken people out of their torpor, people who are well-intentioned but mired down in a system tainted by the attractions of money and power, a system which seems endlessly to snuff out new initiatives that could offer benefits for humanity."

As if he were chorusing the words of John Polanyi, cited at the beginning of the previous chapter, Naessens complained: "Man has almost completely lost the right to think, or to create, outside the norms established by a scientific dictatorship. For over a hundred years, this scientific hegemony, become a trillionaire, has taken deep root throughout the world to the detriment of the health of its populations. This aberrated status in present-day scientific thinking, resisted by a growing number of conscientious researchers, will be overcome only if people as a whole, 'men in the street,' begin to work, peacefully yet with conviction, to smash a medical 'Berlin Wall' erected by vested interests."

The words of Naessens's address, and the nobility of their expression, could well have merited exposure in the Québec press, but it seemed there was not a single journalist willing to put them to print. Yet, at the end of their uttering, Naessens was given a standing ovation.

When the English version of the Canadian edition of my book, which had begun to circulate in the United States, came into the hands of Robert Atkins, M.D., author of two bestsellers on "alternative" health and medical director of the Atkins Center for Complementary Medicine in Manhattan, this widely known physician resolved to do an interview with me on his weeknight radio show, "Design for Living," which is heard by an audience of thousands in an area stretching from New Jersey and eastern Pennsylvania to southern New England.

Atkins began: "Friends, well, tonight we have something very special! Very special! Because we're going to talk about the treatment of cancer, and of other illnesses, by a scientist, a biologist, whose name is Gaston Naessens. We are going to learn about his science and about the results that have been achieved with this remarkable therapy, based on his remarkable discoveries."

It is too bad that the airwaves carrying Atkins's voice could not have reached—in French translation—into Québec province itself, even right into the office, home, or car radio of Augustin Roy himself.

During the interview, Robert Atkins went over with me the highlights of Naessens's findings and their meaning for a new medicine and biology. When I explained that the essence of Naessens's approach was to strengthen the immune system so that it could take care of the body's afflictions, he significantly added: "That's most interesting, because everyone I've ever interviewed, every system I've ever seen that is successful in the treatment of cancer, says just that! Don't destroy the cancer . . . but support the immune system!" What an effect, I thought, would those trenchant words have had if Atkins had been able to speak them at Naessens's trial!

And Atkins did not limit himself to supportive commentary. "I'm planning," he announced to his large radio audience, "to go up to Québec and learn his technique. I know I just *have* to do that because I'm so happy to know that it exists!"

The feedback to the Atkins radio show was impressive. The following day, at the offices of the American Society of Dowsers, in Danville, Vermont, where my book was stocked for sale by mail, over 150 calls were received from a dozen states, asking that it be sent as quickly as possible. Over half a dozen of the calls came from doctors of medicine, among them a physician with his own "alternative" clinic in Norman, Oklahoma, who said he had been invited to go to Los Angeles to be interviewed for a position as a "medical expert" host on a West Coast radio show that goes out all across the nation. If he won the appointment, he said, he wanted to do a second interview with me on Naessens.

Atkins was as good as his word. Within two weeks, he drove, with his attractive Russian wife, Vera, from New York

City to Rock Forest, where he spent the weekend with the Naessenses, learning everything he could about their science — viewing their blood at the microscope and the film made through it — and mastering the technique of injecting the 714-X into the lymph system. Before he left, he told the Naessenses that he wanted to get started on tests with cancer patients.

Upon his return to New York, Atkins devoted a second hour of "Design for Living" to his visit with the Naessenses in Canada. His introductory words could not have been more laudatory:

> I'm here to give a report on what might well be the most exciting development in the history of medicine. Gaston Naessens is surely one of the greatest scientists of the twentieth century. He deserves not just one but several Nobel prizes for his lifework. He probably won't get them, however. Like many other pioneers of alternative cancer cures, he probably will be discredited.

From the southeast tip of the United States, another call came from Roy Kupsinel, M.D., an Ovideo, Florida, physician who edits and publishes *Health Consciousness*, a magazine with the engaging subtitle "A Forum for Accent in Credible Medicine," which goes out all over the world. In a follow-up letter, Kupsinel informed me that he had earlier received my article "In Defense of Gaston Naessens," published in *New Age*, and had been "mighty tempted" to get my okay to reprint it. Instead, he said, he prevailed upon Viktor Penzer, a Polish-born physician and dental surgeon now in his seventies who likes to say that his third diploma — in nutrition — was received from "Auschwitz University," where he had miraculously survived for three long years, to read my book. As a result, Penzer told Kupsinel that he couldn't wait to go up to Rock Forest and interview Naessens for an article in *Health Consciousness*.

Meanwhile, back in Québec, although no doctors had come forward to back Naessens with any declarations as positive as those made public by Atkins and Kupsinel, it nevertheless seemed that a few "waves" were beginning to appear on the French-speaking province's medical waters.

None other than *L'Actualité Medical* (*A.M.*) (The Doctors' Newspaper), had, unbeknownst to Naessens, published a front-page March 1990 article entitled "Alternative Medicine: Where Do Doctors Stand?" This article credited Naessens with having been the main stimulus causing the pot of that debate to start boiling again after a long period of quiescence.

In an interview, the head of the Québec Holistic Medical Association (Q.H.M.A.), Dr. Gilles Vezina, made no bones about a situation in which the potential *recognition* of the merits of alternative medicine was pitted against the determined resistance of the "medical world," an odd euphemism for the medical establishment, particularly its "crowned heads." "Anything new is seen as threatening for those at the apex of medical power," said the president. "Their excuse for their not recognizing alternative medicinals is that there is *no scientific proof* for them. But the reality is that they just don't want to take the trouble to investigate."

Far more shocking was the president's revelation in *A.M.* of the lengths to which the Québec Medical Corporation was going to prevent and block any growth of so-called "holistic medicine." When doctors—and patients—called the corporation's offices to ask how to get hold of the Q.H.M.A., full documentation on which the corporation had been provided, they had been told that *no such organization existed!* It seemed that, just as in the case of Naessens, the medical establishment believed that *lying* to the public was no sin, certainly not a crime. That this attitude is also prevalent in the United States will be documented in the final pages of this book.

Another aspect of the Medical Corporation's "blocking tactics" was revealed when Vezina told the "Doctor's Newspaper" that his formal request that Q.H.M.A. be listed in the corporation's *Annuaire Medical*—a thick handbook listing the names and addresses of all Québécois physicians, as well as all medically affiliated organizations—had been summarily denied.

And even that was not the worst of the situation with regard to the promulgation of alternative medicine in Québec, added Vezina. Speaking for the panel, he made clear that young medical students, avidly interested in alternative medical treatments and techniques, were being offered no help or encouragement whatsoever in their search to obtain information about them.

When, for instance, second-year med students at the University of Sherbrooke's Medical School had asked of its dean that they be allowed to organize on campus a colloquium on "Complementary Medicine," they were categorically refused access to meeting halls, audiovisual equipment, and financial support. The only reason given for the rejection was that the colloquium had nothing to do with the medical school's "teaching curriculum." Unabashed, the students went on to organize the colloquium off campus, by themselves, to organize it, in Vezina's words, "from A to Z." And they were planning another colloquium for the fall of 1990, which, the Q.H.M.A. president was happy to report, this time had won the benediction of the Department for Family Medicine.

It is strange that, by midsummer 1990, neither Dr. Vezina nor any of his Q.H.M.A. adherents had dared to visit with, or even to call, Gaston Naessens. One can only assume that the pressure of the Québec Medical Corporation was effectively blocking any such initiative.

In contrast to that reticence, however, Naessens was most pleased in July to receive a call from Ontario saying that three doctors affiliated with the national Canadian Holistic Medical Association (C.H.M.A.)—all of them young women—would be driving the following day all the way from

Toronto to pay him a call. With them, they brought a specialist in "dark-field microscopy" who had trained with a master
of that technology in Detroit.

During a whole afternoon, much of it spent by the four-
some in looking at blood specimens through Naessens's microscope—in an act of curiosity up to then unmatched by any
Québécois doctor—the group received a virtual "blitz education" in recognizing things they had never seen or been taught
to see.

A letter written by one of the members of the group,
Carolyn F. A. Dean, M.D., provides an account of how a young
open-minded physician reacted to what amounted to one of
the most unusual experiences of her life.

"I never thought I would see such a microscope," Dean
wrote. She went on to write:

> The microscopist in our group told us that the somatids,
> and the other new forms that Naessens had discovered,
> were considered by most specialists to be artifacts. But
> he had no trouble whatever in convincing me, and the
> rest of us, that they were real microbiological entities.
> I have seen, and worked with, many microscopes and
> Naessens's is the most impressive apparatus for view-
> ing live specimens I have ever experienced.
>
> If his microscope were put to wide use, we would
> be able to identify when a person's immune system was
> slowing down and take measures to bring it back to nor-
> mal. The whole world is talking about the immune sys-
> tem without knowing what to do about it. Monsieur
> Naessens has given us enormously important insights
> into this process.

As a result of the visit of the C.H.M.A. group, the following day I received a telephone call from Kingston, Ontario, where, that weekend, the C.H.M.A. was scheduled to

hold its annual meeting at the local university. There I met its president, Leonard Levine, M.D., who graciously found a place for me in the speaking program, so that I could present some of Naessens's story to the assembled audience of physicians and nurses.

What will be the result of this is presently impossible to foretell. The Naessens story is still unfolding, much like the stories told on television, multiepisode dramas, during which audiences are compelled to wait a day, a week, or even longer to see what will happen. As the Italian song has it, "Che Sera Sera." And we can only hope that the Naessens "situation"—comic or tragic, as one might view it—will, in either case, have a triumphant ending. Surrounding this situation, as we have seen, has been a cloud of deceit, and now it is time to take that cloud's larger dimensions and to speculate on whether it can be "busted" out of the sky to admit the sunshine of truth that lies behind it.

Chapter 17
Medical Dissent

*Medical students never get to the stage of asking
questions. Let them ask one and see what happens.
My local university library is divided into two main
sections: the medical library where medics can consult
authoritative textbooks on all branches of medicine; and
the general library for everybody else. Significantly, all
works relating to the sociology of medicine, the critique
of medicine, or medical history belong to the general
library, where medical students will not have to be
exposed to the possibility of reading books that might
actually question the premises of the system in which
they are being trained.*

> Dr. Denis MacEoin, "The Myth of Clinical
> Trials," *Journal of Alternative and
> Complementary Medicine,* August 1990

We recall that *Fusion* editor Maher Jahjah concluded his second article with the words that cancer specialists were now
beginning to admit that chemotherapy treatments were "expedients that destroy the health of patients." Was this really
only a parochial reference to a lamentable situation existing
in his home province where no doctor, thus far, has directly
admitted anything of the sort?

A full seven years before Jahjah penned his words, in
1984, a remarkable, now all-but-forgotten conference, the first
of its kind, was held in Chicago. At that conference, explicitly
entitled "Dissent in Medicine," nine eminent physicians from
all over the United States spoke to an auditorium packed with

their colleagues—as well as the press and public—on rank abuses running rife in their profession.*

The central theme addressed at the conference was the propensity of the nation's medical hierarchy to *lie to the public*. In his opening remarks, Dr. Robert S. Mendelsohn, president of the New Medical Foundation, which encourages and supports "innovative forms of medical education," put his finger on why, how, and where that propensity is given birth. "Doctors are trained from their earliest days in medical school not to share full information with the public," said Mendelsohn. "They learn that if they tell the public the truth about drugs that are being prescribed, people will not take those drugs. Of course, they're right!" How could anyone have put the matter more bluntly?

Equally blunt was Alan S. Levin, M.D., a distinguished professor of immunology at the University of California (San Francisco) Medical School, who rose to protest against the *lies* being perpetrated with respect to cancer treatments. Laying the shocking truth, as he saw it, right on the line, he said acerbically: "Practicing physicians are intimidated into using regimes which they *know do not work*. One of the most glaring examples is chemotherapy, which does not work for the majority of cancers."

Had Levin said as much at the trial of Gaston Naessens, one might well have wondered what reactions to his words would have been evoked in the press, or in the minds of the president of the Québec Medical Corporation or the three cancer specialists who, at their press conference, slammed the door on Naessens's promising treatment.

But Levin did not stop there. Going further he added: "Despite the fact that most physicians *agree* that chemotherapy is largely ineffective, they are *coerced* into using it by

---

*For a complete transcript of the conference, see *Dissent in Medicine: Nine Doctors Speak Out* (Chicago: Contemporary Books, 1985).

special interest groups which have vested interest in the profits of the drug industry."*

On the drug industry's control of cancer therapies, and on its total lack of concern as to whether remedies forced on patients were effective or not, Mendelsohn was even more explicit. "The only proven factor in orthodox therapies," he stated, "are their *adverse reactions*. Doctors not only admit this but are proud of it. According to Eli Lilly, head of the huge drug company which bears his name: '*Any drug without toxic effects is not a drug at all!*'"

Lilly could well have been speaking about Gaston Naessens's 714-X, the completely nontoxic effects of which, as we have seen, have been proven beyond shadow of doubt, as has its effectiveness on hundreds of cases of cancer or other diseases.

As the conference proceeded, it became clearer and clearer that drug dispensers were focused on company *profit* rather than on the succor of patients. It was a distressful fact that "cancer therapies are being oversold," said Dr. George Crile, head of the famed Cleveland Clinic, and that, if appropriate studies were made, doctors "would be led to completely abandon many radical therapies they now use."

What is blocking such "appropriate studies," one might ask, particularly one of 714-X by the Canadian Health Ministry or any other official body?

It was Samuel Epstein, M.D., professor of occupational and environmental medicine at the University of Illinois Medical Center, who gave not only an answer to that question

---

*Full documentation to back up Levin's almost heartrending statement has now been supplied in a thick book, *The Cancer Industry* (New York: Paragon Books, 1990), written by Ralph W. Moss, who resigned from his job as assistant director of public affairs at Sloan-Kettering, one of the world's largest cancer research and treatment centers, to lay the facts before the public.

but provided recommendations as to what helpless citizens, whether cancer victims or not, might do to turn the tide.

Characterizing the whole of the multibillion dollar "phony war" against cancer, declared way back under the presidency of Richard Nixon, as only a "useful paradigm in failed decision making," he was not afraid to state that hundreds of thousands of Americans had died of cancer over the intervening years chiefly due to policies promulgated from on high. His "considered view," added this doctor, was that "there have been no major advances in the treatment of cancer." Far from any battle, not a single skirmish had been won in the war.

Why then, asked Epstein, were legislators in the U.S. Congress uninterruptedly allocating, and justifying, the increasingly immense sums being spent futilely on cancer warriors? His answer? Because they were continually being *lied* to by the "high command"! And Epstein was not loath to target the leading culprits, to single out the "command posts": the American Medical Association, the National Cancer Institute, and the American Cancer Society.

Epstein did not mince words about their actions: "As the public tax dollar has gone to swell their budgets, over the past decade in particular, these institutions *have perpetrated a hoax about our ability to treat and cure cancer* and, at the same time, have fought hard against increasing attention to prevention. We know a great deal about cancer, particularly about how to prevent it. It is my view that what we need now is to *take responsibility for* policy making in cancer prevention away from the institutionalized basis. . . . Instead, decisions should be made with the involvement of the citizens at large of this country. . . . We need a National Citizens' Commission to inquire into the failures of the institutions. We need to *politicize* this issue and remove it from the hallowed corridors of scientific authority."

Epstein's was not the only voice calling not just for dissent, but for action. Echoing that call in the strongest terms, Dr. Levin, in his own closing remarks, felt that only a grassroots political movement could ever overcome the outright prevarication disseminated by the medical dictatorship.

As if he were talking specifically about Gaston Naessens's 714-X treatment, Levin held that ordinary doctors, no less than their patients, were in a "fix" that only a populist mass movement could remedy. His appeal to all laypeople in the Chicago auditorium was a paragon of simplicity: "Your family doctor is *no longer free* to choose the treatment he or she feels is best for you, but must follow the dictates established by physicians whose motives and alliances are such that their decisions may not be in your best interests.

"You the taxpayer, the voter, the consumer, can help stop this corruption. Support your physician if he tells you the *truth* about drugs considered to be the 'standard of practice' in the treatment of a given disease. Support your doctor when he uses *unconventional* modes of treatment which you feel have improved your health. Recognize that he is risking his livelihood and his personal freedom for your well-being."

Could not Dr. Levin have been talking about any physician of the stamp of Michel Fabre, the only doctor in the world to come to testify on Gaston Naessens's behalf in the courtroom drama of 1989?

What was the way out of the mess of authoritarian rule in medicine? Here it is, as Levin proclaimed it over the microphone: "Write to your congressperson or your senator. If your doctor appears to be harassed by the local medical board or the police, remember that that doctor would rather *help you* than comply with the *edicts of the health industry*. With your support, he or she can join the ever increasing number of physicians who have repudiated the *tyranny* of the health industrial complex!"

"Help you . . . rather than comply"—as I typed those words, they seemed, as literally as figuratively, to character-

THE BATTLE CONTINUES

ize the whole of Gaston Naessens's lifelong effort, and to suggest for him an honorary doctorate in medicine so that he could take his place in the ranks of that "ever increasing number of physicians" repudiating "*tyranny.*"

"Thy banners make tyranny tremble . . . "—so runs a line in the patriotic song "Columbia, Gem of the Ocean," learned by most American schoolchildren.

If in 1984 Dr. Levin had raised his banner on high against what he so incisively defined as tyranny, another banner of larger dimensions was unfurled at the start of the last decade of this millennium. Emblazoned with the title "Cancer Manifesto: 1990s," it calls for the overthrow of the "organized, monopolist, autocratic, murderous tyranny known as 'orthodox medical treatment of cancer.'"

Sixteen pages long, it was published in the Winter 1990 issue of the *Newsletter of the Bio-Electro-Magnetics Institute,* a new organization founded by John T. Zimmerman, Ph.D., which has two medical doctors on its board of directors and three more on its advisory board. The author of this remarkable document is Barry Lynes, a science writer who has written three important books on the cancer cover-up.

The new document takes its cue not from the famous Communist Manifesto proclaimed over a century ago, which itself brought about changes as revolutionary as any ever seen in this world, but from a more modern politically inspired one signed by 240 courageous men and women. Issued on 1 January 1977, this manifesto was circulated underground throughout Soviet-dominated Czechoslovakia to prospective supporters as "dissident" with regard to their country's enslaved status as Dr. Levin and his eight fellow speakers were "dissident" with regard to the present enslaved status of the practice of medicine.

Detailing facts about medical skulduggery that can make anyone's hair stand on end, the manifesto enjoins "all those convinced of an evil comparable to totalitarian communism in the form of a medical mafia, *particularly in the treatment of cancer*, to form a civic society in which free citizens take responsibility for their actions."

In so doing, it takes the recommendations of the medically dissenting doctors in Chicago one giant step farther by opening an avenue for people everywhere to express themselves no less decisively than the six women and five men on Gaston Naessens's jury expressed themselves with their ringing verdict.

Lynes feels strongly that, however long it has taken Americans to recognize the horror of what has been going on in its cancer wards, many of them with "human radar tuned to the nightmare that is cancer" are becoming awakened and can be mobilized into a countervailing force.

That a lone individual can contribute to this force is exemplified in Lynes's manifesto by the case of a man who recently took out a full-page advertisement in his local newspaper attacking the cancer establishment. A letter, one of dozens, received by this man, gives an idea of the very horror of the "system" that is cancerology:

My best friend died of breast cancer four years ago. She was, of course, subject to the same scenario you have portrayed. Her last months were spent being herded, with others, like cattle through radiation treatments, where women were lined up without privacy and "zapped" by the machine. She was then started on chemotherapy, which made her last days sheer hell. As she lay dying, a directive came from a doctor requesting a scan and other expensive tests, *all to be performed within the last six hours of her life*. At that point, her husband ordered everyone away from her and let her have her remaining time in peace, no longer just a human experiment.

Which of us, reading these lines, cannot believe that the woman had entered a torture chamber as ghastly as any that can be conceived? Or compare, in his or her mind, the descriptions of a "peaceful dying" provided earlier in this text, when patients given 714-X, even if they could not be saved, were allowed to pass away in tranquility?

What is the nature or substance of the "killing instinct" of doctors who continue to administer treatments that, as Dr. Levin put it, *they know will not work*? As I was writing these lines, I received a call from an associate in California, one of whose close friends had just been "put to death" by zealots operating a radiation device. The really sad part of this tale is that the man, diagnosed with lung cancer, had begun to take Naessens's 714-X and was seen to be responding *most positively* to the treatment. Yet radiation, in what turned out to be a massive overdose, was nevertheless continued. It caused such terrible burns on his body that, unable to recover from them, he died. My associate was told by one of the doctors on the hospital staff, who could not prevent the radiation from taking place, that it alone was responsible for the man's death. He never had a chance to find out if, like so many others, his life could have been extended by Naessens's product.

It is because of hundreds of cases similar to the two just described that Lynes writes in his manifesto: "Let us never again permit such unrestrained power to abuse innocent patients or scientific innovators."

What can the individual do? Here is Lynes's answer: "On a personal level, what is asked of you is very little. The next time you go into a hospital cancer ward or a cancer clinic and witness the bottles suspended from hooks above patients' heads, sending poisonous liquids into their bodies, recognize you are in buildings created by criminals.

"Next time you hear such titles as the Mayo Clinic (Minnesota), the Sloan-Kettering Cancer Center (New York), the

M. D. Anderson Cancer Center (Texas), or any of the many others, or the National Cancer Institute, the American Cancer Society, the U.S. Food and Drug Administration, the Board of Quality Assurance, or your own local medical society, don't just silently let the conversation proceed about the way cancer is conventionally treated. Stop it right there, and challenge it! That's your moment of truth. Be political, be outspoken. Stand up!

"Inform people around you about the crimes initiated and still supported by those in charge of all such institutions and their ilk. Even if you are resented by your friends for disturbing their comfortable world, no matter. Keep in mind that what you are denouncing is no less than a 'party headquarters' of a tyranny no different from the one being dismantled in Eastern Europe and the Soviet Union."

Confident that his "call to arms" will succeed, Lynes ends with Winston Churchill's dictum that "the United States of America is the mightiest force in the world and can remain so. When that nation is united in a righteous cause, it will prevail *over all evil interests.*"

If some would regard Barry Lynes's "Cancer Manifesto," as utopian, they might nevertheless warm to a prediction that, due to what amounts in our country to a medical crisis of increasing proportions, orthodox medical hegemony will be forced to abdicate its throne as a result of its no longer being able to cope with its responsibilities.

This is the view of Dennis Stillings, director of the Archaeus Project in Saint Paul, Minnesota, which promotes new concepts in biomedicine such as "cyberbiology," or the effects mind can have upon body that are crucial to self-healing. In July 1990, Stillings spoke before the annual meeting of the U.S. Psychotronics Association, of which he was, at the time, president. Referring to an appalling increase in degenerative disease, Stillings stressed that the current situation in that regard has become so desperate as to now be ushering the notion of *rationing* into the field of health care. "We have reached a state wherein medicine, as traditionally practiced, is in a near state of collapse because of its astronomically rising costs," said Stillings. "Part of the problem is not to be laid at the feet of overworked doctors but at the door of ecological systems, both outer and inner, those of the earth itself and of the organisms that walk upon it, that are under mounting invasion by a host of enemies, recognized and unrecognized."*

If, due to the expanding breakdown in immune systems, the medical profession has to confess an inability to cope with a tidal wave of patients, Stillings was of the opinion that its rulers will necessarily have to forfeit the right to dictate to people what kind of medical care they are allowed to have, or not allowed to have. And, as he saw it, this will, in turn, open the way to the inevitable erosion of power of medical "associations" and "corporations" of all kinds, as well as that of such regulatory bodies as the U.S. Food and Drug Administration and all the rest of the authoritarian organizations listed by Lynes in his manifesto. At that point, "alternate" medical approaches could become as legally valid, and competitive, as orthodox ones.

Stillings sees the "Naessens Affair" as vitally central to this issue. As he wrote to me: "I want to pay special atten-

---

*At the Chicago conference, Dr. Epstein, anticipating Stillings, referred to the twentieth century as being one of "major threats to society, which stem from 'runaway technology' in the hands of expert *'idiot savants,'* whose rate of progress has been so rapid as to outstrip the capacity of social control mechanisms. One of these threats is the chemical industries' role in 'carcinogenizing' our environment with a wide range of toxic chemicals, thus contaminating our air, water, food, and workplaces, as well as hazardous waste dumps all over the country." He might have well added the *soil itself*, in which most of our food is grown (see *Secrets of the Soil* by Peter Tompkins and Christopher Bird, New York: Harper & Row, 1990).

tion to Naessens's ongoing story since, up to now at least, it represents *the* model of an 'outsider' going against mainstream medicine with a demonstrably effective treatment. Such an apparently *clear-cut case* is rare."

Will the "cancer tyranny" have to cede its ground to new brilliant approaches such as those of Gaston Naessens, as implied in Stillings's scenario? Opinions differ, and there are some that are hardly optimistic. One dour conclusion is that of Frederick I. Scott, Jr., a veteran commentator on "frontier science" who has for years written hard-hitting editorials on that topic for the widely distributed magazine *American Biotechnical Laboratory*. Devoting one of his editorials to Naessens and his work in the August 1990 issue of that magazine, Scott positively began:

> While the courtroom may be the last place one expects to find scientific enlightenment, dramatic challenges to scientific dogma played out there can profoundly influence the course of science in application and teaching. This is particularly true in the case of so emotionally laden a disease as cancer. The trial of Gaston Naessens in Québec, Canada, from November to December 1989, may prove to be of such profound influence for it broaches issues of fundamental perceptions in microbiology and microscopy.

Even though he knew nothing about it, Scott thus seems to support Canadian attorney Peter Weldon's assessment of the Naessens trial.

However, in the conclusion to his piece—which masterfully presents the Naessens saga to his scientifically trained readers—Scott turns less sanguine. Expressing strong doubts that any "people power" can ever break a "scientific paradigm" that bars the existence of fundamentally new ideas into its practice, he writes:

There is little basis for that belief. We simply cannot afford it. We have livelihoods and long-standing prestigious careers invested in *what exists.* These are in control of what, in that paradigm, is to evolve. Nothing in our training or circumstances provides any mechanism by which we can examine or implement such ideas without devastating personal, professional and, more importantly, financial consequences.

And a further communication from bacteriologist Walter Clifford, in a single of many possible examples, illustrates why Scott may have every right to be so pessimistic. Clifford writes to the director of an organization that gives a prestigious annual international award to individuals who have substantially contributed to rewrighting (as in "shipwright") our disrupted ecologies, inner and outer, everywhere.

"I am honored to offer comment concerning the work of Gaston Naessens," he begins. Then, in no uncertain terms:

> You are quite correct that there are numerous quarters which would rise in revolt if an award were presented to this gifted and noble scholar. However, their ignorance and bigotry do not negate the truth nor the value of Naessens's contributions. I recall an occasion before I met Naessens when a respected pathologist sat with me at the microscope so that he might be shown the peculiar microbiology of the blood. After nearly an hour of looking at a specimen of his *own blood,* he arose and walked out of my office. When I called out to him as to why he was so upset, he indicated that he *did not believe what he had seen!*

And Clifford ends with a "punch line" that may well justify Scott's black outlook: "His last comment was to the effect that if he were to acknowledge what he had seen, *his*

*professional colleagues would turn against him and cause
him to lose a valuable practice.* So much for professional
objectivity."

Given this report, how can Scott, and many, many others,
not have deep misgivings that the yearnings of all people will
eventually overcome the selfish motivations confronting
them? Can Scott be right in so lugubrious a conclusion? In
other words, is the paradigm Thomas Kuhn described, in the
medical sense, secure? Or can personal commitment, as called
for by Barry Lynes, finally shift, or break, that paradigm? Are
human cultural developments basically *outside* human control, leaving us at the mercy of an evolutionary juggernaut,
the course of which is predetermined by influences about
which we have neither any real knowledge or mastery?*

Just as I was finishing this book in early September 1990,
I had the opportunity to address the 18th Annual Conven-
tion of the Cancer Control Society in Pasadena, California.
The society is a citizens' group made up of cancer victims—
many of them who have recovered due to "alternative" treatments that shore up deficient immune systems, such as that
of Gaston Naessens—enlightened medical doctors, and laypeople. In addition to delving into nontoxic cancer therapies

---

*Readers given to pondering such questions should consult one of
the few books that has left a permanently disturbing imprint on
me since I read it many years ago. Wholly displeasing to those who
purportedly believe they are "in charge" of our destiny, and purport
to be able to "run" our affairs, *The Science of Culture* (New York:
Farrar, Straus & Giroux, 1969), by anthropologist Leslie White, maintains that human "culture," in its widest aspects, is a "creature" with
a life of its own, totally unresponsive to human desires and, therefore, control. The book asks a fundamental question, the very one
asked by Thomas Kuhn: "Do changes take place at a *time* propitious
for their changing?" Or, as Shakespeare put it: "There is a tide in
the affairs of men, when taken at the flood, leads on . . . to victory. . . ." How much longer will the vessel of Gaston Naessens's
discoveries have to wait for "flood tide"?

and nutritional approaches to the prevention of cancer, the society also provides valuable information on legal aspects of the rights of individuals to choose what they consider best for themselves in the field of medical treatment.

Before giving the audience a rundown on Naessens's discoveries and achievements—including his smashing court victory, which has put him in the world spotlight—I couldn't resist citing some passages from a book that had come to my attention the day before. Among others, the book quotes a congressman from the state of Iowa who announced: "The medical monopoly is not only the meanest ever organized, but one of the greatest dangers that has ever menaced a free people."

If members of the audience could easily have believed those words might have been printed in either the transcript of the 1984 Chicago "Medical Dissent" meeting, in Barry Lynes's "Cancer Manifesto 1990s," or in Ralph Moss's new book, *The Cancer Industry*, that impression was further reinforced by another of the book's statements: "The medical doctor's craft has become a complete tyranny and the public put into its permanent slavery which is enforced by the power of state and federal law."

Most exciting to the audience, however, was one of the same book's ringing predictions: "Of late, various drugless healing systems have become so numerous and strong, and the old school of medicine has been suffering the loss of people's confidence to such an extent that it is only a question of a very short time and the old medical camp will be completely deserted."

The audience sat rapt as they heard that prediction seemingly promising victory in a virtual "civil war" in the medical field and imminent emancipation for the "slaves." Unable to stand the suspense, one man heaved himself out of his chair to ask me for the title of the book containing the passages I had just read.

"Can you, or anyone else here, guess the names of the book's title and its author?" I countered.

Several contemporary books on the question of the treatment of cancer and the "politics" surrounding it were mentioned.

"It may come as a disappointment to you," I said, almost impishly, after the guesses had been made, "but I have to tell you that the title of the book in question which runs nearly six hundred pages, is *The Medical Question: The Truth About Medicine and Why We Must Have Medical Freedom*. It was written by a Dr. A. A. Erz, a naturopath and chiropractor, and published by another doctor, Benedict Lust, in a Florida town called Tangerine. Its date of publication—1914, or nearly seventy-five years ago!"

That being the case, it might seem that Frederick Scott, Jr.'s gloomy prognostics are not so far off the mark.

Yet what are all of us to do in the face of this injustice? Are we simply to become resigned to a status quo, or an existing "paradigm"? Or do we take the same kind of action that the Québec Committee for the Defense of Gaston Naessens took in the summer of 1989, action that mobilized provincial, national, and international backing for a literally unknown pioneer, action that may well have tipped the juridical scales in his favor?

This is a question that was squarely posed in a communiqué received two days following the Cancer Control Society's conference. It was issued by the research institute run by a physician and biochemist Stanislaw Burzynski, in Houston, Texas. The institute's claim is to have discovered certain biochemical compounds and derivations in the human body that, when administered intravenously or orally, are capable of restoring cancer cells to normalcy.

The effectiveness of the treatments is exemplified by the case, reported in the communiqué, of a little eight-year-old boy, Jimmy, diagnosed with terminal brain cancer, whose mother was told that nothing more could be done to save him. At her wit's end, she brought her son in a wheelchair to Burzynski's clinic on 4 January 1990. By mid-August, the patient had abandoned the wheelchair and was, in the communiqué's words: "very close to complete remission."

Then, in a cry of alarm, the same communiqué reported on a concerted effort by three separate bodies—the U.S. government (Justice Department), the Texas State Board of Medical Examiners, and, strangest of all, the insurance behemoth Aetna—to close down Burzynski's treatment center.

This latest effort was only the most recent in a long series of harassments designed to put the Texas doctor out of business. One such attempt, in 1983, mounted by the Federal Food and Drug Administration, resulted in a court ruling that he could continue his practices only if they were limited to the state of Texas and not exported beyond its borders. In the interim, Burzynski provided the FDA with so much documentation on the success of his treatments that, if piled in a single stack on the floor, it would reach higher than the topmost hair on the head of a person six feet tall.

So now, it turned out, the Texas medical "rulers," joined by the U.S. government and insurance interests, were resolutely trying to plug the "loophole" through which a United States court had allowed Burzynski to practice, at least in his home state.

The new action, as the communiqué made horrifyingly clear, was taken not just against a doctor and his research institute, but against *patients* who, because ninety percent of them sought Burzynski's help only *after* they had been told they had no other options, stood to lose more than Burzynski himself.

"Our government's action is literally against Jimmy, and many others like him," wrote Le Trombetta, the research institute's director for public information, who told me over the telephone that Burzynski's legal fees had been running over $100,000 a month!

Explaining that the latest tactic of the U.S. Justice Department was to indict Burzynski criminally on mail fraud charges, Trombetta, bringing Barry Lynes's general recommendations into specific focus, continued: "We have the power to generate the *two things* that government agencies most fear: a congressional investigation, and adverse publicity. Our strength is in our numbers and in the truth behind what we're doing."

Trombetta listed a number of pointed questions to help Burzynski's would-be supporters formulate exactly what they should ask representatives in Congress to look into. Among them were:

> *Whom* does the government claim to be protecting in its action?
>
> If the protection is not for patients, since they have not requested it, then is it for a *private interest group*, and at the risk of those patients' lives?
>
> *Who* are the key players, inside or outside the government, pushing to close down Burzynski's operation? *What* do they stand to gain by eliminating his nontoxic treatment?

We have seen that questions of this kind were, in the main, answered in Naessens's case, by the trial reported in this book. Whether Burzynski's own trial will provide answers remains to be seen. And it may be that only a trial can provide them.

A fifty-page chapter, "The Fiercest Battle," on the Burzynski case, in Moss's *The Cancer Industry*, provides other interesting parallels between the outlooks of the Texas doctor and the Québécois biologist and the methods used to distort and dismiss their findings.

To his attackers, writes Moss, "Burzynski is a clever opportunist, exploiting a mysterious and ineffective cancer 'cure' of his own imagining. His treatment is bizarre, expensive, useless and also possibly dangerous." Were not these the same allegations and accusations made with respect to Naessens by the Québec Medical Corporation and the three cancer specialists who held the press conference in Montréal?

Moss continues: "But to his patients and supporters, Burzynski is a gentle physician who has saved or prolonged hundreds of lives with his innovative approach. . . . In addition, he really cares about their well-being in an old-fashioned way rarely seen in today's oncology clinics." This is no less than what Naessens's own patients and members of his defense committee have said about the biologist both in public and in court.

There is still another tie between the two cases, a tie suggesting that Canada, far from becoming more liberal in its attitude toward promising cancer treatments, only reflects the rigid opinions of the cancer hierarchy in the United States. As far back as 1982, two Toronto doctors were named by the Ontario Medical Association to go to Texas and investigate Burzynski's treatment. Though their travel to Houston took the better part of a whole day, their review of his voluminous records lasted no more than two hours, or not even as long as the short time Dr. Jolivet had spent with Naessens.

In their highly critical report, they accused Burzynski of keeping the nature of his products "secret," which was no more or less than what Augustin Roy had repeatedly said of Naessens. But far from being secretive, Burzynski, says Moss, attempted to explain all his production techniques to the two doctors in great detail. Just as Naessens had and has explained his to Dr. Jan Merta de Velehrad and anyone else who would listen.

Furthermore, Moss notes that Burzynski was given time to show the visiting doctors records of only nine cases before they decided to leave. Of the nine, six had obtained *complete remission* of cancer and two nearly complete remission.

And, as in the case of Naessens's 714-X, the doctors also tried to dismiss the effectiveness of Burzynski's treatments by alleging that it had been made only after the patients had been treated by orthodox means. In fact, only one of the nine cases had received radiation and chemotherapy.

When Burzynski urged the two Canadians to look at more cases, they refused. And when he suggested they take a pile of them back to Canada and examine them at their leisure, they also refused. "They were," said Burzynski, "very anxious to leave the clinic as soon as possible." Yet, when they returned to Canada, they were able to write a report saying they had not a single positive thing to say about Burzynski's treatment. And, going one step further, they strongly recommended *against* any insurance reimbursement for treatments at his clinic.

Most significant in all this is Moss's statement that the comments of the two Canadian doctors, widely circulated not only in Canada itself, but in the United States, "soon became the touchstone of opposition to Burzynski."

Whatever the outcome of Burzynski's forthcoming trial, his public relations director, Le Trombetta, recommended in her communiqué that, in the case of her boss, the "time had come to investigate the investigators." Since this could only be done by Congress, she urged Byrzynski's adherents to mobilize as many letters as possible to their state representatives in Washington, D.C., as well as to Burzynski's own congressman and to members of both the House and Senate Judiciary Committees. "We must ask the question Jimmy's mother has asked," she concluded: *"How do they dare?"*

Was all this just "whistling in the dark"? Or can actions by citizens turn a tide? It is left to readers of this book to decide and, if the answer to the second question is *yes*, to act.

As for Le Trombetta, she closed her communiqué with an opinion offered by the renowned anthropologist and author, Margaret Mead: "Never doubt that a small group of thoughtful, committed citizens can change the world. Indeed it's the only thing that ever has."*

---

*Another example of an initiative taken by a private citizen is that of Conrad LeBeau, owner of Vital Health Products, in Muskegon, Wisconsin. LeBeau has started a movement to end fifty years of government-controlled medical monopoly by unleashing the power of the Ninth Amendment to the U.S. Constitution. This little known amendment reads: "The enumeration in the Constitution, of certain rights, shall not be construed to deny or disparage others retained by the people." LeBeau has issued a "Ninth Amendment Legal Defense Kit," the use of which, he maintains, can lead to practical steps to win freedom of choice in medicine and health care, one of the rights retained by the people under the amendment.

LeBeau has also reprinted an interesting book, *The Forgotten Ninth Amendment: A Call for Legislative and Judicial Recognition of Rights Under Social Conditions of Today*, by Bennett B. Patterson of the Texas Bar (Indianapolis, Indiana: Bobbs-Merrill, 1955). Mr. Patterson writes in his conclusion: "The Ninth Amendment to our Constitution is a guarantee of our individual personality. . . . May all of us be humbly grateful to a Creator who has endowed us with a soul, and a constitutional government which guarantees to us the right to own it." (The materials can be obtained from Vital Health Products Ltd., Box 164, Muskegon, WI 53150).

Chapter 18
Epilogue: An "Enemy of the People"

Now, as the lights dim in the universities and much of the most exciting intellectual activity goes on outside of academe, the time seems right to recognize, and encourage, independent scholarship. . . . Where do new ideas come from, which ignite thousands, sometimes millions of people? Most often, they come from the work of one independent, brilliant, driven thinker or investigator.

Ronald Gross, *Independent Scholar's Handbook*

As the summer solstice grew closer and the daylight hours were becoming the year's longest, the Montréal *Gazette* announced the screening of one of "the best teledramas made over the last twenty years," a new production of Norwegian playwright Henrik Ibsen's masterpiece *An Enemy of the People*. In that stage play, written over a hundred years ago, the only doctor in a small coastal community discovers that the waters in its highly lucrative spa, visited by countless wealthy clients, have been contaminated with a lethal form of bacteria.

When the doctor alerts the community leaders to the danger, his warning is venomously rejected by all of them, including the mayor, the doctor's own brother. To suppress the truth, they begin a concerted campaign to destroy the doctor's reputation and credibility. By the time their campaign is over, not only has the physician become a reviled outcast in the society he has so loyally served, but his wife and children find themselves ostracized by their friends, neighbors, and playmates. As I watched the stirring story un-

259

fold, it came to me that Ibsen's theme was just as valid today as it was when he addressed it a century ago.

If Naessens had been branded in his own community
as a people's enemy, there were hopeful signs that many of
those "people" were solidly behind him. When the biologist
came to the Baron Hotel to deliver some materials to me,
several persons, attending a rock concert in its garden, surged
out of a large crowd to shake his hand and offer congratulations, as did passers-by in the streets and shops of Sherbrooke.

As if they had read and been inspired by Barry Lynes's
manifesto, patients who had completely recovered their
health following 714-X treatment were engaged in various
"political" strategies. One young man, who had put Hodgkin's
disease behind him, took the trouble to call Marc Yvan-Côté,
Québec province's minister of health, to say he owed his life
to Naessens.

To his surprise, instead of rebuffing the former cancer
victim, the minister entertained a long conversation with
him, during which he asked the caller what *he* thought should
be done to change the medical climate in the province. When
the patient replied that, first and foremost, legislation to make
alternative medical practices permissible, and available,
should be enacted, the patient was startled to hear the minister at least partially agreeing with his suggestion.

On the other hand, the case of the wife of a prominent
Québécois political leader, as it relates to Frederick Scott's
gloomy conclusions, reveals how "careerism" controls individuals in the most desperate straits. In the final stages of
lung cancer, this woman, though aware that 714-X might be
her salvation, refused to have it clandestinely administered
for fear that, were her treatment with the product to become
publicly known, it might gravely injure her husband's political career, even bring it to an end.

But, at the same time, Gerald Godin, whose brain cancer
seemed, at the very least, to have been arrested in its progress,

was heard by thousands of Québécois citizens, during a summer television interview, to declare that he had "nothing but respect" for Gaston Naessens.

If certain tokens of popular support seemed to be heralding a rosier future for Naessens, truly significant evidence that his fortunes were changing for the better began to manifest in the waning days of August. Mounting professional interest, not only in his treatment modes but in the whole of his *Nu* biology, began to appear as suddenly as a sun breaking through a heavy layer of clouds. Into the darkness shrouding Québec poured light rays from Europe and the United States.

One searchlight penetrating the gloom was Christoph Gisler, Ph.D., a biochemist who heads up Bio-Galenic, named for the famous Greek physician Galen, a "Center for Biomedical and Orthomolecular Information" in Geneva, Switzerland, which publishes *Orthomed-Letters.*

As explained in one of Gisler's broadsides, the word *ortho*, in Greek, means "adequate," "fitting," "correct," or simply "good." Why Gisler, who had read a copy of the Canadian version of this book, had made the long journey to Rock Forest is revealed by a passage in the same broadside: "Orthomolecular medicine derives from well-established biomedical research and uses therapeutic techniques and preventative practices. It can be summed up as: a comprehension of biochemical mechanisms in the body and the utilization of nontoxic substances, harmless to the body, to create conditions of optimal health." Was it any wonder why the Swiss biochemist was excited by 714-X, which, if anything, was certainly "orthomolecular."

The handsome and affable Gisler was in no mood to waste time. He began with a visit to the Canadian publisher

---

*For many years, Gisler was scientific director for the Upjohn laboratories.

of this book to order two hundred copies for display at an international exposition of orthomolecular medical products sponsored in Geneva in October 1990 by Aquarius, a French-language publishing house with which Gisler's center has affiliation.

During a day's conversation with the Naessenses, Gisler told them that orthomolecular practice was burgeoning so fast all over Europe—largely due to popular demand for it—that pharmacists were in *a race* to offer their customers effective new products exactly like 714-X, and drug companies were gearing up to make them available. Gisler knew what he was talking about, if only because his contacts in the pharmaceutical field include Georges Marti, father of Gisler's pharmacist wife, Françoise, who is owner of Galencia S.A. in Zurich, the largest pharmaceutical firm in Switzerland.

Before he left for the airport to return home, Gisler signed an agreement for the exclusive right to distribute Naessens's intralymphatically injected medicinal in his own country as well as in France, Italy, Germany, and Austria, with options for the Iberian peninsula and the United Kingdom.*
On 12 September, Gisler declared in writing that his collaboration had three aims: to spread the news on the benefits of 714-X (and other products developed by Naessens); to make them easily accessible to doctors, so that patients could profit from them; and to advance Naessens's research on all fronts.

If Gisler's visit was for Gaston Naessens the equivalent

---

*Those with international connections, which many American and Canadian researchers lack, are apparently making "end runs" around a virtual dam blocking the development and distribution of new medical products in North America. While confronting a pincer movement designed to immobilize him in Texas, Dr. Stanislaw Burzynski has been able to get a Swiss pharmaceutical firm to export his anticancer product for trial in Japan, after the U.S. Food and Drug Administration not only tried to discourage the Japanese from testing it, but refused to allow its export from the United States.

of a sunrise in the east, shortly after the departure of the Swiss, more "suns" seemed to be peeping over the southern horizon. A flurry of phone calls from south of the border testified that American medical men and women who had learned of Naessens, through publicity circulating ever more widely about the Canadian edition of this book, had, to use Gerald Godin's words, "nothing but respect" for the biologist's achievements.

Taken aback by the surge of interest and the broad scope of questions coming in over their telephone line, the Naessenses, realizing that they could not handle the queries on a one-by-one basis, decided to organize an impromptu seminar in Rock Forest so that all concerned could convene there to hear, and compare notes on, what would be presented at it.

Over the first weekend in September, a group of medical practitioners made the long journey to the Eastern Townships. Among them were five M.D.s from Massachusetts, Connecticut, New Jersey, Pennsylvania, and California; an optometrist from Florida; two chiropractors from Virginia and Pennsylvania; and a dentist from Connecticut; as well as a man practicing nutritional medicine from Ohio and two nurses from unspecified American cities.

Most of them had been mobilized by microbiologist Walter Clifford, who constantly travels around the whole of the United States to consult with medical practitioners. His own remarks at the meeting brilliantly introduced the whole group to the significance of Naessens's discoveries. The rest arrived as a result of their having independently heard of Naessens's work through the "grapevine" and consequently having called him to get more information.

Proceedings got underway on a Friday, in an auditorium at Sherbrooke's Delta Hotel, where, with the help of a professional interpreter Daniel Tessier, Naessens gave a long "retrospective" of his life work, going all the way back to the development of his first cancer products in France. Various articles, both in French and English, were read aloud in their original versions or in translation, and interrupted by many questions from the fascinated visitors.

Particularly interesting to the assembled crowd was one written by John W. Mattingly, inventor of the world-famous "Water Pik," a water-pressured "toothbrush" for home use, and an adjunct professor of the philosophy of science at Colorado State University. The paper outlined in detail the whole history of the Pasteur-Béchamp controversy and decades-long attempts by researchers to understand the nature and effects of polymorphic organisms in the blood, all the result of Mattingly's extended and devoted independent study of the topics.

Present at the seminar was expert microscopist Dr. Bernard Grad, a retired professor of biology at McGill University, who had learned his microscopic art during his student days from none other than Dr. Wilhelm Reich, at whose research center, Organon, in Rangeley, Maine, Grad had spent hundreds of hours in training. A few months prior to the seminar, Grad had visited Naessens's laboratory to spend several hours observing various specimens through the microscope, during which time I heard him declare that he was viewing structures in detail that he had never before seen, a professional opinion he also shared with the seminar's participants.

The next day, Saturday, the whole group, enlarged to a total of twenty-five with the arrival of several of Naessens's relatives and guests, crowded, like a herd of horses in an undersized corral, into the small house and even tinier laboratory, virtually packing the latter from wall to wall. There, for the first time in their lives, the American visitors were able to view somatids in their own blood and many of the aberrant pathogens in the sixteen-stage cycle in the blood of a cancer patient, all through Naessens's somatoscope.

One could easily say that, over the course of Naessens's long career, never, in a single day, had so much been seen by so many medical specialists.

The general consensus, as expressed by several doctors

present, was that all of them had seen a body of work providing a *completely new direction* in science and in medicine, and had been privileged to hear, for the very first time, a *fully coherent presentation* of the complexities of the cycle of microbes in the blood, especially because it incorporated a lucid explanation of how that cycle originated with the somatid. That "coherence" had been, for the most part, achieved by the screening on television of Naessens's thirty-eight-minute film made at the microscope and his "voice-over" commentaries. Many of the doctors asked for copies of the cassette to show to their colleagues when they returned home.

The properties of the somatid and its apparent effects on genetic systems, as well as its ability to block *rejection* of skin grafts in animals, were highly startling to the assembled medicos, for whom most of Naessens's findings amounted to "brand new territory." Over the telephone, I received comments from three of them, which ran as follows:

It was just tremendous . . . the whole scope of it . . . to be able to see so many new things and talk to people who had had firsthand experience with 714-X, which seems almost like a "magic bullet." I'm most excited about what I saw, and heard, and have read in your book, a copy of which I bought when I was up there in Québec. I'm certainly going to recommend that book to many people and I'm going to recommend the treatment to people I know who need it.

Every member of the group was nothing short of awestruck! How one man has been able to place in total human perspective things that most people are literally unable to conceive. I believe Gaston Naessens should receive a Nobel prize in science and another for peace, as well, because of what he has done for the welfare of humanity. Now the task is to get the "news" out in "low-

key" fashion, which will bring Gaston the recognition
he so richly deserves.

I was really impressed with Naessens's knowledge and
the scientific evidence I saw to back it up. So impressed
that I immediately ordered a $20,000 Zeiss research mi-
croscope so I could see some of the things he has been
seeing. In his microscope, I saw many things I've never
before seen and I have done microscopic work for a long
time. I think it may be a long time before Gaston's
findings are accepted, because they'll be resisted to the
end by those who don't believe, or don't want to believe,
them. But there are a lot of "freethinkers" out there and
if we can get them to use Naessens's technology, that
will be a way to win acceptance for him.

The seminar, it turns out, may be a harbinger of many
more to come, inasmuch as many of its participants, before
taking their leave, suggested to Naessens that they had colleagues just as avid as they themselves to see and hear everything to which they had been exposed. And, almost every day,
Naessens and his wife are receiving more calls from the
United States to inquire when they can come to Québec to
visit him. It is becoming clear that the next symposium may
well attract over two hundred persons. To prepare for it, Naessens is envisioning the publication of an illustrated handbook
presenting the entire substance of his research and answering the kinds of questions asked at the first seminar.

Another no less interesting result of the seminar was
a change in course in Naessens's thinking with respect to the
future development and distribution of his unique microscopic technology. While, prior to the time of the seminar's
convening, the biologist had planned to improve his existing
instrument and make it available at a cost of some $100,000,
he was led to alter this view. Recognizing that doctors, such

as the ones who had made the effort to come all the way to Rock Forest, were in need of an affordable microscopic tool, he became convinced that he could adapt standard "dark-field" microscopes, with which most of them are familiar, so that these can clearly reveal all phases of the somatid cycle.

If this can, in fact, be done, it will allow for instruments costing in the neighborhood of only $10,000 to be placed in the hands of biomedical scientists unable to afford a microscope costing ten times that amount. In this way, the whole array of Naessens's findings could become widely disseminated, and his years-long isolation brought to an end.

It was indeed fortuitous that all this European and American support came when it did. For Naessens's troubles with the law are still not over. The Rock Forest researcher is awaiting another trial for "illegal practice of medicine." This time the case involves two medical double agents, or "spies," working for the Québec Medical Corporation. In 1989, they visited Naessens under assumed names with "phony" complaints. When he was kind enough to examine their blood and inform them that they could not have the afflictions they said they had, their only thanks was to report him for having performed a "medical service" contravening established statute, which led to his citation. Naessens knew beforehand what might be afoot, because one of the spies was so unprofessional in her undercover work that she wrote, under the rubric "Home Address" in his daybook, the address of the Québec Medical Corporation itself.

The good news in this regard is that the third trial, scheduled for May 1991, may not take place. This is because legislation currently pending in Québec's parliament, if passed, will prevent the Medical Corporation from continuing its base practice of using agents to spy on private citizens. Naessens's defense lawyer, Conrad Chapdelaine, is hopeful, even fairly confident, that the charges will be dropped, in which case Naessens may never again have to tread the steps of a courthouse.

Yet it also appears that the Medical Corporation is by no means giving up its malicious campaign against Naessens. In fact, it is extending it to assault his allies. In September 1990, just prior to the seminar, the biologist received an overseas call from Dr. Michel Fabre in France, who had had the courage to appear at his 1989 trial as the only doctor of medicine willing to testify in Naessens's defense. Incredible as it may seem, Fabre reported that an investigation of his activities had begun in France *at the demand* of the Québec Medical Corporation, which had asked the French medical association to launch it. The investigation centered on whether Fabre might be "psychologically unbalanced," given his testimony at the trial at which, reported the Québec Medical Corporation to its French counterpart, Naessens *had been found guilty!* Partly due to that bald-faced *lie,* Fabre was threatened with suspension of his medical license. But he affirmed to Naessens that he had no intention to stop treating patients with 714-X and that Christoph Gisler's Bio-Galenic center in Switzerland had entered the fray to support him.

Given all these new developments, positive and negative, pro and con, what does the future hold for Gaston Naessens? One thing is nearly certain: Naessens is out in the limelight to stay. And he does not necessarily relish that kind of prominence.

His chief aspiration is to establish a research body to repeat objectively all of his experiments and get them written up in language acceptable for publication in journals of science. This will require the full-time assistance of several bright, young "postdoc" specialists—as able and eager as Daniel Y. E. Perey—in a number of disciplines. Naessens also hopes that his new assistants will be able to answer many questions about aspects of his discoveries that have so far eluded explanation.

Work already done must be pushed farther. To take only one example, the exchange of somatids from one animal to another must be studied. Not only do the effects of this exchange open a virtual "Pandora's box" in the science of life, but if it can be determined that such exchange would permit organ transplants *without rejection syndromes*, that, in itself, would be a biomedical finding of staggering proportions. The facts are there for all to see. Surely there are young researchers who have the vision.

To attract backing for the research program as just outlined, the Naessenses have set up a Fondation UNIVERS (Universe Foundation), the capitalized French acronym standing for the "National Union for Investigation, Validation and Experimentation in Scientific Research." It hopes to raise several millions dollars.

Finally, while his new assistants are working on the validation of his former research, Gaston Naessens wants to liberate himself from all other responsibilities to the point where he will be able, as before, to begin *brand new* research based on long formulated, and more recently formulated, ideas. To have, in Canadian Nobel Laureate Polanyi's words, "the freedom to pursue truth whereever it may lead." Or, as Dr. Jan Merta de Velehrad put it: "to get on with life's central aim, the search for valid information."

All people of goodwill wish Gaston Naessens well in his aspirations. They are asked for their help, and that of their friends and associates: help for the discoverer of the somatid, not an "enemy," but a true friend, of the people.

Appendix A

What Has Become of the Rife Microscope?

by Christoper Bird
Originally published in
New Age Journal *(March 1976)*

This article, like an embryo or any living thing, is still growing. A continuum of this growth may depend upon the assistance of NAJ readers, their colleagues, and their friends.

Originally I intended to write a short note on what was known about the Rife microscope. Precious little is in print on the subject.

One day, while waiting for some material to come up from the cellar stacks of the National Library of Medicine in Bethesda, Maryland, considerably frustrated by the lack of leads and data concerning the demise of the Rife microscope, I wandered by the Subject card catalogue and casually flipped at random to a card in the middle of a drawer labeled "Microscopes."

The card was filed under "Allied Industries," as if that firm was the author. The company's address was stated to be 4246 Pepper Drive, San Diego, California. The title referenced was "History of the Development of a Successful Treatment for Cancer and Other Virus, Bacteria, and Fungi."

At the bottom of the card was a single line: "Written by Dr. R. R. Rife."

Entirely by accident, I had stumbled upon what looked to be only one of a series of reports written by Royal Raymond Rife. Fourteen pages long, it was numbered Dev-1042. It was approved and signed by I. F. Crane, manager; Don Tully, development associate; and Verne Thompson, chief electrical engineer.

Are any of these gentlemen alive today?

Was Allied Industries a research corporation established by Rife?

How many other reports did it publish and where are they?

The report so riveted my attention that I was compelled to explore some of the history of microbiology and its connection to cancer and other disease. The present article, much longer than originally planned, is thus the result of a fortuitous finding—perhaps an example of what Jung has called *synchronicity*—and the consequent preliminary exploration.

Much more needs to be done to tell the story of Rife and his microscope, a fascinating episode in the history of science.

The Microscope of Microscopes

In February 1944, the Franklin Institute of Philadelphia published an article, "The New Microscopes," in its prestigious journal devoted to applied science. Founded in 1824 by "philosopher-mechanics," the institute, which recently made studies in its physics laboratory on the best way to move the Liberty Bell to its new Bicentennial Year location, is a smaller analogue of the huge world-famous Smithsonian Institution in Washington, D.C., which reprinted the same article in its own journal shortly after its first appearance.

Authored by R. E. Seidel, M.D., a Philadelphia physician and his research assistant, M. Elizabeth Winter, the essay opened with a six-page discussion of the electron microscope, which had only recently been put on the market by the Radio Corporation of America. This microscope is today standard equipment in modern laboratories.

The article closed with a ten-page treatment of a "Universal Microscope," the brainchild of a San Diego autodidact,

Royal Raymond Rife, who developed it with the financial assistance of the rollerbearing and axle magnate Henry H. Timken, for whose family Rife at one time served as handyman and chauffeur.

Rife's scope, the largest model of which consisted of 5,682 parts and required a large bench to accommodate it, overcame the greatest disadvantage of the electron microscope, its inability—because tiny living organisms put in it are in vacuum and subject to protoplasmic changes induced by a virtual hailstorm of electrons—to reveal specimens in their natural living state.

With his invention, Rife was able to look at living organisms. What he saw convinced him that germs could not be the cause, but the result, of disease; that, depending on its state, the body could convert a harmless bacterium into a lethal pathogen; that such pathogens could be instantly killed, each by a specific frequency of light; and that cells, regarded as the irreducible building blocks of living matter, are actually composed of smaller cells, themselves made up of even smaller cells, this process continuing with higher and higher magnification in a sixteen-step, stage-by-stage journey into the micro-beyond.

Though, with the aid of Rife's device, thousands of still pictures and hundreds of feet of movie films were made to reveal these facts, all of this material and the Rife microscopes seem to have disappeared without a trace.

Or have they?

Calls to the U.S. Armed Forces Institute of Pathology Medical Museum, which has hundreds of different microscopes in its historical collection, to the National Library of Medicine's Historical Division, to the Smithsonian Institution and the Franklin Institute (both repositories for outstanding scientific inventions) and to a dozen establishments dealing daily in microscopy elicited from curators, medical pathologists, physicians, and other scientific specialists only the complaint that none of them had ever heard of Royal Raymond Rife and his microscope.

What has become of the Rife microscope?

The question is not rhetorical. For if even half of the possibilities described for this astounding discovery are true, a massive effort to hunt it down and reactivate its potential might not only save billions of dollars in biological and medical research but open a fascinating new vista onto the nature of life.

From the start, Rife's main goal was to find cures for disease, especially the most intractable of all diseases, cancer. Because he had a hunch that some as yet undiscovered microorganism would prove to play a crucial role in the onset of this malignancy, he tried unsuccessfully to find one by observing all types of malignant tissue with a variety of standard research microscopes.

In the 1920s it became obvious to Rife that a better means of scrutinizing the microworld than had been developed was indispensable. During that decade, he designed and built five microscopes with a range from 5,000 to 50,000 diameters at a time when the best laboratory microscopes in use could achieve not more than 2,000 diameters of magnification.

At the Rife Research Laboratory on Point Loma, California, he worked at magnifications of 17,000 and higher, to reveal a host of cells and microorganisms never before seen and to photograph them. The work required a saint's patience. It could take the best part of a day to bring a single target specimen into focus.

The Rife microscope had several arresting features. Its entire optical system of fourteen lenses and prisms, as well as an illuminating unit, were made of crystal quartz, which is transparent to ultraviolet radiation. In the scope, light was bent and polarized in such a way that a specimen could be illuminated by extremely narrow parts of the whole spectrum, one part at a time, and even by a single frequency of light.

Rife maintained that he could thus select a specific frequency, or frequencies, of light that coordinated and resonated with a specimen's chemical constituents so that a given specimen would *emit its own light* of a characteristic and unique color. Specimens could be easily identified, thus solving one of microscopy's greatest bugaboos. It was *control of illumination* that turned the trick.

Another feature was the microscope's extraordinary resolution, its ability to reveal the most minute of component parts of any specimen so that each may be seen distinctly and separately from the others. Imagine two extremely thin parallel lines. When they can be clearly distinguished, you are still within the microscope's range of resolution. If the parallel lines blur together, high magnification will only enlarge the distortion and limit of resolution has been attained. With a resolving power of 31,000 diameters—as against 2,000 to 2,500 for the laboratory microscopes in common use in that day—Rife's device could focus clearly on five lines of standardized grid, whereas an ordinary microscope could do no better than examine fifty lines, and that with considerable aberration. This is somewhat equivalent to one aerial camera's being able to spot individual houses in city blocks from a very great height, while another is able only fuzzily to distinguish the single city blocks themselves.

Controversial Discoveries

Beginning in the 1920s and continuing over seven years, Rife and his colleagues worked on more than 20,000 laboratory cultures of cancer obtained from the Paradise Valley Sanitarium in National City, California, in what appeared at first to be a fruitless effort to isolate microorganisms that he felt should somehow be associated with the disease.

Up until then, bacteria had clearly been proven to be linked with a wide variety of ills including tuberculosis, leprosy, cholera, gonorrhea, syphilis, typhoid, bubonic plague, pneumonia, and others. But no one had found them in association with cancer.

In contrast to the much smaller viruses, bacteria were widely considered to be unicellular, monomorphic (meaning one shape and one shape only) forms. A quarter of a million of them can occupy a space no larger than the period at the end of this sentence. They come in various shapes. Cocci are round, bacilli rodlike, to offer two examples.

There are various forms for each shape. Of the round-shaped ones, monococci appear singly, diplococci come in pairs, staphylococci in clusters resembling a bunch of grapes, streptococci, which under certain conditions can produce a painful sore throat, in chains.

While outside a host, or body, bacteria are hard to raise, or culture. Each type has been studied as a pure culture type by isolating it upon a specific nutrient called media.

Bacteria also have specific maximum, minimum, and optimum temperatures in which they will live and multiply. Some, like polar bears, are addicted to arctic temperatures and even live in ice. Others prefer water so hot it would kill most animals. A great many enjoy the temperature of the human body. Millions of them are living, harmlessly, inside you right now.

But they are not always harmless. They can acquire virulence, or the power to cause disease, under some conditions but not others, although even today no one knows exactly why.

This mystery, in the 1920s, was closely connected to a debate in microbiology so hot as to seem almost a war. On one side were those who affirmed—as do many textbooks today—that bacteria were *eternally monomorphic.* They could not assume other or smaller forms, as small, say, as a virus.

Originally, *virus*—the word means "poison" in Latin— was the name generally applied to any microscopic agent injurious to living cells. Now it is much more narrowly defined as "one of a unique group of very small infectious agents that *grow only in cells* of animals (including humans), plants, and also bacteria."

Because they were so small, viruses would pass through filters that did not allow the passage of bacteria, said to be monomorphic, just as a net of small enough mesh will allow minnows to pass through it but bring the fish that are preying upon them up short. It is this filter-passing ability of viruses that is widely held today—along with their inability to grow on artificial media—to be one of the main criteria separating them from bacteria.

For several decades, however, another school of microbiologists maintained that, far from holding everlastingly to one shape, bacteria were *pleomorphic*, or form changing. They could be caused, under the right conditions of culture, to metamorphose into forms small enough to pass through filters just like viruses.

Because of their sharp disagreement on the filterability of bacteria, the two camps came to be called "filtrationist" and "nonfiltrationist."

One of the earliest of the filtrationists was a Swedish physician and explorer, Ernst Bernhard Almquist, for whom islands off the north Siberian coast are named. Almquist made hundreds of observations of pleomorphic bacteria in his laboratory as did researchers in Italy, Russia, France, Germany, and the United States. In 1922, after two decades of work, Almquist came to the conclusion that "nobody can pretend to know the complete life cycle and all the varieties of even a single bacterial species. It would be an assumption to think so."

Way back in 1914, the American bacteriologist Dr. Edward C. Rosenow had the gall to assert that bacteria were *not* unalterable and that various strains, or what one might call sub-subspecies of them, could, when suitably treated, become any of the other strains. It was Rosenow's contention, too, that he found a form of the streptococcus bacterium which caused poliomyelitis, commonly known as infantile paralysis.

What Rife's opinions were about this heated controversy are not known. He followed the standard bacteriological practice of the day, first implanting small patches of cancer tissues on various nutritive media including a special "K" medium developed by another filtrationist, Dr. Arthur Isaac Kendall, at the Northwestern University School of Medicine in Chicago, Illinois. The medium, which bore the first letter of Kendall's name, seemed to have the faculty of transforming bacteria into the transitional forms alleged for them by the filtrationist school. No matter how often he changed menus for his sought-after cancer microbe, no matter how he altered the temperature of incubation, Rife seemed unable to coax it to appear in his cultures.

It was apparently only when, as a result of his continuing physical experimentation with the effects of light frequencies, he discovered that many microbes respond to the effects of light from noble gases, such as neon, xenon, and argon, by changing their growth patterns that Rife hit upon a solution to the problem that was nagging him.

He placed a sealed test tube containing cancer tissue into a closed loop filled with argon gas. After creating a vacuum within the loop, he charged the gas with electricity, just as one does when one throws the switch to light up the neon lamps in modern offices, though in Rife's case the charge was 5,000 volts. While he still could not reveal any microbes, he noted a certain cloudiness in the nutritive medium, which, through chemical analysis, he ascribed to ionization caused by the electronic bombardment.

Readers may well wonder *why* he adopted so strange and novel a process. The question is just as unaswerable as if put about Rife's next step: In order, he said, to counter the ionization, he placed the tube into a two-inch water vacuum and heated it for twenty-four hours at near body temperature.

Under his microscope, at 20,000 X, the tube now teemed with animated forms measuring only 1/20 by 1/15 of a micron—much smaller than any known bacteria. They refracted a purplish red color in the specific light beam.

He called this form Bacillus X and, later, because it was so much smaller than other bacilli, and perhaps because of the filterability controversy, BX virus. This problem of nomenclature can be resolved herein by referring to Rife's organism as a BX form, or simply BX.

Rife writes that "this method of ionization and oxidation brought the chemical refraction of BX out of the ultraviolet and into the visible band of the spectrum. Owing to the fact that the test-tube specimens had gone through so many trials, we again started from scratch and repeated this method 104 consecutive times with identical results."

Because he could culture his BX form, so small it would pass through any filter, he seemed to have discovered a *filterable form* of a bacterium. But just finding bacteria, even in filterable form, in a human tumor does not necessarily imply that they are its cause. To make sure, it is held they must be reinjected into animals and seen to cause the same or nearly similar disease, after which they must then be reisolated and shown to resemble the original organism. These were the postulates propounded by the German pioneer bacteriologist Robert Koch, who proved that tuberculosis was apparently caused by the tubercule bacillus.

Following this accepted procedure, Rife inoculated the new BX forms into over 400 rats in all of which there subsequently appeared "tumors with all the true pathology of neoplastic tissue."

Some of the tumors became so large they exceeded the total weight of the individual rats in which they were developing. When the tumors were surgically removed, the BX form was recovered from them in all cases. Koch's postulates were fulfilled.

More Startling Discoveries

By continued microscopical study and repeated photography to stop their motion, Rife and his co-workers next came to the baffling conclusion that the BX, far from remaining always what he had seen as the purplish red bodies a fraction of a micron in dimension, could change into not just fairly similar forms as Rosenow had previously discovered, but into *completely different forms* simply by altering the medium on which they were living only very slightly.

"Slightly" in Rife's case meant an alteration in the nutrient environment of only two parts per million by volume. Those who would consider this unlikely may recall that in homeopathic medicine doses of remedies are given in dilutions of this weakness and beyond. Even though they have nothing chemically analyzable in them, they are effective.

One such alteration caused the BX to become what Rife called a Bacillus Y, or BY. It was still the same purplish red color as the BX but so enlarged that it *would not* pass through a filter.

With the second change of the medium, the BY enlarged still further into a monococcoid or single disk form which, when properly stained, could be viewed under a standard research microscope. Rife claimed that these forms could be found in the blood of over ninety percent of cancer victims.

By removing this form from the fluid medium it inhabited and depositing it onto a hard base of asparagus or tomato agar, Rife then saw it miraculously develop into a fungus, making it kin to a yeast, mold, or mushroom.

Any of these succeeding forms, Rife stated, could be *changed back* within thirty-six hours into a BX form capable of producing cancer tumors in experimental animals from which, in turn, the same BX form could again be recovered.

The transformation did not stop with the fungus, which, if allowed to stand dormantly as a stock culture for a year and then replanted onto the asparagus medium, would then *change into bacillus coli,* millions of which live in the human intestine. This common bacillus could pass, in Rife's words, "any known laboratory method of analysis."

Because he had found that microorganisms had the ability to luminate when stimulated by given frequencies of light, it occurred to Rife that they might also be *devitalized* by beaming radiations of specific frequencies upon them. One source has it that the harmonics of these frequencies ranged from 10 meters to 20,000 meters.

To this end, he had been developing concurrently with his microscopic equipment a special frequency emitter, which he continued to improve, up to at least 1953, as steady advances in electronics continued. The killing waves were projected through a tube filled with helium gas and said to be efficient in destroying microorganisms at a distance of as much as one thousand feet.

With this device, he noted that when the proper mortal oscillatory rate was reached, many lethal organisms such as those of tuberculosis, typhoid, leprosy, hoof-and-mouth disease, and others appeared to disintegrate or "blow up" in the field of his microscope. This "death ray" principle was also effective when applied to cultured BX.

The obvious next step was to determine whether similar radiation would affect the BX, not in culture, but in the bodies of cancer-afflicted animals. It apparently did so, for Rife states he got rid of BX in over 400 experimental rats and other animals in his lab. If it worked on animal cancers, wondered Rife, why not on human cancers?

The answer was so resoundingly "Yes" that, in our day when billions are being spent each year to find a cure for cancer, it is prudent to quote Rife's report word-for-word:

The first clinical work on cancer was completed under the supervision of Milbank Johnson, M.D., which was set up under a special medical research committee of the University of Southern California. Sixteen cases were treated at the clinic for many types of malignancy. After three months, fourteen of these so-called hopeless cases were signed off as clinically cured by a staff of five medical doctors and Alvin G. Foord, M.D., pathologist for the group. The treatments consisted of three minutes duration, using the frequency instrument which was set on the mortal oscillatory rate for BX, or cancer, at three-day intervals. It was found that the elapsed time between treatments attains better results than cases treated daily.

The News Leaks Out

News of Rife's work began to leak out to the world of medicine at the end of the 1920s. One of the first to learn of it was Arthur W. Yale, M.D., who lived in San Diego, not far from Rife's laboratory. He acquired a frequency emitter and began to treat cancerous patients.

In 1940, reporting to his fellow physicians on some of his decade-long results, Yale wrote that because the whole of Rife's extraordinary findings constituted an "entirely new theory of the origin and cause of cancer, and the treatment and results have been so unique and unbelievable," he was making his findings available in the hope that "after further research we may eliminate the second largest cause of deaths in the United States."

Yale had had limited success in treating cancerous tumors with X rays and with the use of what he called "static wave current" for some three decades. When he began to use Rife's device, he sometimes employed it alone, sometimes together, with the two methods with which he was familiar. Both methods brought startlingly successful results. Yale was careful to note that, when he added the use of the Rife ray to his other radiation, cancerous masses "have disappeared in about one-tenth the time and so far with no reoccurrences."

Dr. Arthur Isaac Kendall, whose "K" medium Rife had used in his experimentation, was also determined to check whether viable bacteria in the filterable state could be unequivocally seen by Rife's microscope. Kendall had been working with cultures of typhoid bacillus and, under a standard microscope, had been able to detect a swarm of active granules that could be seen only as tiny motile points. Because nothing of their individual structure could be ascertained, Kendall could not diagnose them with certainty to be filterable forms of the bacillus.

In order to make certain, he went to California in late November of 1931 and examined his cultures under a Rife microscope at 5,000 diameters in the Pathological Laboratory of the Pasadena Hospital. The facilities were afforded through the offices of the same Drs. Johnson and Foord who had worked with Rife on the BX.

When Rife finally got them in focus, the tiny granules were seen to be bright, highly motile, turquoise-blue bodies, which, to quote the report he coauthored with Kendall, "constrasted strikingly both in color and in their active motion with the noncolored debris of the medium." The same observations were repeated eight separate times, the complete absence of similar bodies in uninoculated control media being noted.

To further confirm their findings, Rife and Kendall next examined eighteen-hour-old specially cultured and inoculated colonies of the same bacillus because they had determined that it was *precisely at this stage* of growth that they became filterable. Now they could see *three* transitional forms of the same organism: one, the normal bacillus itself, almost devoid of color; two, the same bacillus but with a prominent turquoise blue granule at one end of it; and three, the same turquoise blue granules moving about independently.

This was somewhat equivalent to being able to observe

a caterpillar, its cocoon, and the butterfly that emerges from the cocoon, all simultaneously.

When they transplanted the filter-passing granules into a broth medium, they were seen under the Rife microscope to *revert back* to their original bacillus, or rodlike, form.

At this juncture, the American bellwether journal *Science* got wind of Kendall's work and, in a news story devoted to it, referred to the new "supermicroscope" invented by Royal Raymond Rife. The same month, December 1931, the Rife-Kendall account was published in *California and Western Medicine,* the official mouthpiece of the state medical associations of California, Nevada, and Utah. This magazine also commented editorially that the Kendall-Rife article was to be particularly recommended to its readers because of its "calling the attention of the world to a new type of microscope which, if it fulfills its apparent advantages over any microscope thus far developed, bids fair to lay the basis for revolutionary discoveries in bacteriology and the allied sciences."

The editorial was significantly entitled "Is a New Field About to Be Opened in the Science of Bacteriology?" Apparently it was about to die aborning.

The Opposition Mounts

The following month, Kendall was invited to give the De Lamar lecture at the Johns Hopkins University School of Hygiene and Public Health in Baltimore, Maryland, before the Association of American Physicians. As a leader of the filtrationist school, he attracted the attention of his adversaries, two of whom were invited as discussants.

The first was an irascible, pugnacious curmudgeon, Dr. Thomas Rivers, of the well-heeled Rockefeller Institute of New York City, who was described by one of his institute colleagues as a "difficult and formidable person to oppose and [he] could be stubbornly inflexible in maintaining a position."

When he learned of his invitation to discuss Kendall's

presentation of the work with the typhoid bacillus, Rivers hurriedly repeated experiments on which Kendall had worked for years and, by his own account, got no proof of Kendall's claim. Based on this thin evidence, he arose at the Johns Hopkins meeting and, to quote him, "in a very temperate manner called the fellow a liar. Not in so many words. Actually, all I said was that I couldn't repeat this experiment and I therefore didn't believe his findings were true."

Rivers was followed in the discussion by the Harvard microbiologist, Dr. Hans Zinsser, also a "nonfiltrationist," who, to quote Rivers anew, "just gave Kendall bloody hell. I'd never seen Hans so hot in my life. I had to agree with everything he said—but I really felt sorry for poor old Kendall—he just sat there and took it."

In the midst of the venom and acerbity, the only colleague to come to Kendall's aid was the grand old man of bacteriology, and first teacher of the subject in the United States, Dr. William H. "Popsy" Welch, who evidently looked upon Kendall's work with some regard.

What is of interest today is that at the Baltimore meeting there seemed to be no mention of the Rife microscope. Also, in the light of the apparent victory of the "nonfiltrationists" over those who claimed that bacteria were filterable, it was curious that Rivers could claim to have repeated Kendall's work without the use of the instrument Kendall had found so necessary to clearly reveal his filterable forms.

Kendall's work, however, attracted the rapt attention of the same Dr. Edward C. Rosenow who, in 1914, had been able to prove that strains of streptococcus were able, under the right conditions, to transmute one into the other. In that day, he had written that these "conditions were more or less obscure. They seem to call forth new or latent energies which were previously not manifest and which now have gained the ascendency."

As a filtrationist, Rosenow was a maverick among bacteriologists up to his death at ninety-four in the 1960s. His work had convinced him, also prior to World War I, that organisms in sera—the fluids from tissues of immunized animals commonly used as antitoxins to neutralize microbes in the body—might in some patients have dangerous biological side effects.

The main implication of Rosenow's work in his own eyes was that bacteria were not as important to disease as the terrain on which they found themselves. "It would seem," he wrote in his 1914 article, "that focal infections are no longer to be looked upon merely as a place of entrance of bacteria but as a place where *conditions are favorable for them to acquire the properties* which give them a wide range of affinities for various structures."

Rosenow first became aware of the Rife technique through a patient at the Mayo Clinic in Rochester, Minnesota, where Rosenow was employed. The patient was none other than the same Henry H. Timken, who had financially aided Rife to develop his microscope and begin his research in the 1920s.

Rife came to Chicago with his microscope. Kendall invited Rosenow down to the Northwestern University Medical School to work with himself and Rife on 5 July 1932. For three days, they made a restudy of the Kendall forms, Rosenow working with a Zeiss microscope, Kendall with an oil immersion dark-field instrument, and Rife with his special device. "The oval, motile, turquoise blue bodies," wrote Rosenow of this work, "described previously by Kendall and Rife were unmistakably demonstrated."

The three next decided to filter cultures of the streptococcus bacteria that Rosenow had found to be associated with poliomyelitis to see what the Rife scope might reveal. What they saw were not the blue bodies linked to the typhoid bacillus, but cocci and diplococci of a brownish gray color each surrounded by a strange halo. These could only be observed in the Rife microscope.

Moreover, filtrates of a virus considered to be the cause of encephalitis showed a considerable number of round forms, singly and in pairs, which under the special Rife illumination were pale pink in color and somewhat smaller than those seen in the poliomyelitis preparations.

Rosenow's work was panned by Rivers in public forum just as viciously as was Kendall's. This was *before* Rosenow had worked with the Rife microscope. "I had one run-in with him," said Rivers, "at a meeting held before the Association for Research in Nervous and Mental Diseases during Christmas week in 1931. I was pretty savage with him. Do you think that helped? Hell, no, if you ask me for my candid opinion, I think that most of the audience believed Rosenow."

This belief did not last for long. For a variety of reasons, including the very difficult methods of culturing the filterable forms of bacteria—and lack of the Rife microscope to observe them—the "church" of nonfiltrationist bacteriology, of which Rivers was later proclaimed "the apostolic father" (does one need better evidence of hierarchical priesthoods and priestcraft in science?), was putting the filtrationist camp on the defensive.

Three filtrationists, writing of discoveries similar to those of Kendall, just prior to Kendall's Johns Hopkins lecture, thus considered it necessary to state in their introduction: "It has come about these days that to express convictions that differ from the *consensus gentium* becomes almost professional foolhardiness: It brings down the strictures of one's friends and enemies alike."

They added: "But we are also conscious of the fact that, beneath the tumult of controversy between monomorphism and pleomorphism, there is being born a new epoch in bacteriology, the limits of the significance of which and the possible expansion of which no one can yet surmise."

Like all scientific revolutions, the epoch would have to wait patiently for its time to come. Rosenow was held by his adversaries to be *100 percent wrong* in many of his observations. His son, Dr. Edward C. Rosenow, Jr., chief administrative officer of the American College of Physicians, asserts that his father was all but accused by Rockefeller Institute research moguls of experimental dishonesty.

How was it that none of Kendall's or Rosenow's attackers bothered to use the Rife microscope? Rife himself admitted that he was not confident that his experiments, revealing the BX form, could ever be repeated without the use of his scope. "We do not expect any laboratory," he wrote, "to be able to produce the BX on account of the technique involved and adequate optical equipment. This is why we have never publicly announced that BX is the cause of cancer but we have succeeded in producing from its inoculation tumors with all the true characteristics and pathology of neoplastic tissue from which we have repeatedly recovered the BX virus."

At the end of his life, Rosenow was philosophic about lack of acceptance for his findings among his colleagues. "There is no way," he told his son, "to convince one's peer group of something new until their attitude of receptivity changes. They simply won't listen." This echoes the German Nobel Laureate in physics Max Planck, who stated that for new ideas to be accepted, one had to wait for a generation of scientists to die off and a new one to replace it.

The Search Continues

With respect to Rife's cancer observations, it may be that this process of replacement is now taking place.

Rife's work has a possible connection with research performed over the last twenty years by several pioneers. One pair of them are Dr. Irene Diller, a former long-time associate of the Institute for Cancer Research in Philadelphia, and Dr. Florence B. Seibert, professor emeritus of biochemistry, University of Pennsylvania.

One day in the late 1950s, Diller called Seibert, who won

many awards and five honorary doctorates for her more than thirty-year-long work on tuberculosis, and asked her to come and look at some microbes on slides. On the slides, Seibert observed tiny round organisms. When Seibert learned that Diller had isolated them regularly from many other tumors, as well as from the blood of leukemia patients, she hastened to ask whether Diller could find them in a sarcoma tumor she, Seibert, was studying.

After several weeks, Diller showed Seibert a tube filled with a slightly grayish and moist-looking culture filled with small round cocci. Injected into mice, they produced cancerous tumors.

Seibert became convinced that Diller might have found a link to cancer. Because so many scientists, believing Diller's new forms to be merely "ubiquitous contaminants" in her cultures, were writing off her work as spurious, Seibert decided to continue working on the problem during her Florida retirement, first at the Mound Park—today the Bay Front—Hospital in Saint Petersburg, later at a Veterans Administration Hospital.

Blood samples from cancer patients with varying types of leukemia were obtained and from every one of them Seibert was able to isolate pleomorphic microbes. These bacterial forms were also isolated from tumors, and with an homologous vaccine they decreased tumors in mice. Just like those of the Rife-Kendall-Rosenow research, they could change from round to rod shaped and even could become long threadlike filaments, depending on what medium they were grown in and for how long. They would pass a filter and *at this stage* in their life cycle they were about the same size as Rife's BX forms.

Today there is great stir about, and much money devoted to, viruses in relation to the cancer problem. The most recent edition of the *Encyclopedia Britannica* states that "sufficient evidence has been acquired to indicate that one or more viruses probably cause cancer in man," and that carcinogens, or cancer-producing agents, "are suspected of producing cancers by activating viruses latent in the body."

But, so far, little support is given to those who ascribe bacteria and the forms into which they transmute the ability for close association with cancer. This legacy of the nonfiltrationist school persists in the face of mounting evidence that the filtrationists may have been right all along.

These days, because various bacterial forms have been noted to have anomalies in their cellular walls—how could they develop into smaller forms if they could not leap beyond or through the walls that imprison them? They are known as Cell Wall Deficient Forms. A revolutionary new book about them has been written by the Wayne State University microbiologist Dr. Lida H. Mattman. Her text opens with the statement: "Clandestine, almost unrecognizable, polymorphous bacterial growth seems to occur as often as the stereotyped classical boxcars of bacilli and pearls of cocci. . . ." The book's contents would seem to indicate that the new era predicted in 1931 for filtrationist microbiology is dawning, though presently its adherents are having great difficulty both in publishing their work and getting grants for further research.

Sufficient data, writes Mattman, have been amassed to warrant reinvestigation, and adds: "There is no subject generally viewed with greater skepticism than an association between bacteria and human cancer. However, the medical profession may look back with irony at the stony reception given by his home colleagues to Koch's paper elucidating the etiology of tuberculosis. Similarly, medical students were once taught that whooping cough vaccination was an unrealistic dream reported only by two women at the Michigan Public Health Laboratories and by a pediatrician namer Sauer."

Most importantly, she concludes: "One must always consider that most malignancies are accompanied by an immunodeficiency. . . . Therefore, we could be dealing with a microbe that finds such a host *merely a suitable environment for habitation."*

This is very close to Rife's own statement that he had unequivocally demonstrated that "it was the chemical constituents and chemical radicals of an organism which enacted upon the *unbalanced cell metabolism* of the human body to produce disease." Before he died, Rife stated: "We have in many instances produced all the symptoms of a disease chemically in experimental animals without the inoculation of any virus or bacteria into their tissues."

What, then, of Royal Raymond Rife and his microscope?

Lingering Questions

How is it that biologists and physicians, other than Kendall and Rosenow, did not rush to investigate it? Why haven't physicists looked into the effects Rife achieved with electromagnetic waves of specific frequencies upon disease, including cancer?

Similar effects were observed by Dr. Georges Lakhovsky in Paris, who developed a wave emitter called a multiwave oscillator with which he cured cancer as well as other diseases in plants and humans. The multiwave oscillator is today banned by the FDA as quackery. They have also been noted in Bordeaux by another inventor, self-taught as was Rife, Antoine Priore, whose apparatus combines the use of electromagnetic radiation with a plasma of helium or noble gases reminiscent of Rife's method used in detecting and devitalizing BX.

Are the strange blue, motile forms that Dr. Wilhelm Reich discovered in the late 1930s and for which he coined the word *bions* related to the foregoing? Reich observed the bions to spontaneously proliferate from specially treated organic matter and even from coal and sand! Spontaneous generation of life was supposed to have been laid to rest in Reich's time, as it is in ours, and he was accused by fellow scientists of confusing Brownian movement of subcellular particles or debris in his cultures with the new subcellular forms he claimed to have discovered.

In cancerous patients, Reich observed the bions to degenerate into what he called T-bacilli (the T coming from the German word *Tod,* meaning death). When injected into mice, they caused cancer just like Rife's BX forms.

In Copenhagen, a biophysicist named Scott Hill reports that a new book written in Russian by two researchers at the Kazakh State University in the U.S.S.R. deals with a whole new branch of medical science in which "healing" of various disorders is being accomplished by the use of ultraweak, monochromatic laser light. Shades of Rife!

The Lee Foundation for Nutritional Research in Milwaukee, Wisconsin, maintains that Rife, his microscope, and his life work were tabooed by leaders in the U.S. medical profession and that any medical doctor who made use of his practical discoveries was stripped of his privileges as a member of the local medical society.

Rife himself died three or four years ago. Considerable digging has not established what happened to his estate. The remarkable instrument he conceived and developed and its photographic evidence may still be in existence. They are worth looking for.

The assistance of *NAJ* readers is solicited.*

References

Seidel, R. E., and M. Elizabeth Winter. "The New Microscopes," *Journal of the Franklin Institute,* February 1944.

---

*After the above article was published, further investigation located Rife's "Universal Microscope" in a sorry state of disrepair in the San Diego home of John Crane. Efforts to rebuild it have so far been unsuccessful. A fascinating book on Rife's saga, *The Cancer Cure That Worked,* by Barry Lynes, was published in 1987 by Marcus Books, Toronto, Canada.

Allied Industries, "History of the Development of a Success-ful Treatment for Cancer and Other Virus, Bacteria and Fungi," Report no. DEV-1042, 1 December 1953, written by Dr. R. R. Rife.

Rosenow, E. C. "Transmutations Within the Streptococcus-Pneumococcus Group," *Journal of Infectious Diseases*, vol. 14, 1914.

Rosenow, E. C. "Observations on Filter-Passing Forms of Eber-thella Typhi (Bacillus Typhosus) and of the Streptococcus From Poliomyelitis," Proceedings of the Staff Meetings of the Mayo Clinic, 13 July 1932.

Yale, Arthur W. "Cancer," *Pacific Coast Journal of Homo-ecopathy*, July 1940.

"Filterable Bodies Seen With the Rife Microscope," Science Supplement, *Science*, 11 December 1931.

"Is a New Field About to Be Opened in the Science of Bac-teriology?" Editorial, *California and Western Medicine*, December 1931.

Kendall, Arthur Isaac, and Royal Raymond Rife. "Observa-tions on Bacillus Typhosus in its Filterable State," *Califor-nia and Western Medicine*, December 1931.

Kendall, Arthur Isaac. "The Filtration of Bacteria," *Science*, 18 March 1932.

Almquist, E. *Biologische Forshungen Weber die Bakterien* (Biological Research on Bacteria), Stockholm, 1925.

Benison, Saul, and Tom Rivers. "Reflections on a Life in Medi-cine and Science," an oral history memoir prepared by MIT Press, 1967.

Hadley, Philip, Edna Dalves, and John Klimel. "The Filter-able Forms of Bacteria," *Journal of Infectious Diseases*, vol. 48, 1931.

Seibert, Florence B. *Pebbles on the Hill of a Scientist*, self-published, Saint Petersburg, Florida, 1968.

Mattman, Lida H. *Cell Wall Deficient Forms*. Cleveland, Ohio: CRC Press, 1974.

Greenberg, Daniel S. "The French Concoction," *Esquire*, July 1975 (full account of Antoine Price and his invention).

Lakhovsky, Georges. *La Formation Neoplastique et le Desequilibre Oscillatoire Cellulaire* (Neoplastic Formation and Cellular Oscillatory Disequilibrium). Paris: G. Doin, 1932.

Reich, Wilhelm. *The Cancer Biopathy*. New York: Orgone Press, 1948.

"The Rife Microscope of 'Facts and Their Fats,'" Reprint no. 47, The Lee Foundation for Nutritional Research, Milwaukee, Wisconsin.

Inyushin, V. M., and P. R. Chakorov. *Biostimulation Through Laser Radiation and Bioplasma*. Kazakh State University, U.S.S.R. (in Russian).

Diller, Irene. "Tumor Incidence in ICR-Albino and C37/B16JN-icr Male Mice Injected With Cultured Forms From Mouse Malignant Tissues," *Growth*, vol. 38, 1974, page 507.

Seibert, F. B., F. M. Feldmann, R. L. Davis, and I. S. Richmond, "Morphological, Biological, and Immunological Studies on Isolates From Tumors and Leukemic Bloods," *Annals of the New York Academy of Sciences*, vol. 174, 1970.

Seibert, F. B., "Decrease in Spontaneous Tumors by Vaccinating C3H Mice With an Homologous Bacterial Vaccine," *International Research Communications Service*, vol. 1, 1973.

Appendix B

714-X: A Highly Promising Nontoxic Treatment for Cancer and Other Immune Deficiencies

by Gaston Naessens, Biologist

When one views cancer as a cellular disease, isolated from general biological disorders and developing along proper norms that are local and independent of any possible carcinogenic agent whose persistence is no longer indispensable to the autonomous progression of the tumoral process, the therapy is centered on "the tumoral mass," whose destruction and radical removal becomes the only imperative means of recovery.

Until now, among the means at our disposal for combating this disease, the surgical solution has figured most prominently. This solution, which best addresses the notion of "tumor as a local disorder," consists of the radical removal ofthe autonomous and parasitic mass from the cellular agglomeration, which appears as an immediately palliative solution.

Next came the radiation solution. This therapy applied to tumors, which proposes the destruction of the tumoral mass by deep disintegration of the cancerous cells and for which the question of dosage and irradiated surface is an important consideration, would not be efficient other than to the extent in which the radiation would reach the neoplastic cells, not with the intent of immediate and blind disintegra-

Reprinted by permission of the author.

tion but rather to force a reversal of the pathological synthesis that is the source of their malignancy.

Finally came the chemotherapeutic solution. The therapeutic solution based on the use of chemicals toxic to such cells, which is to say by karyoclasic poisons that stop the mitoses by plasmatic division and chromatic alteration, leads to duplications of the number of chromosomes and abnormal mitoses. The karyoclasic action of this therapy appears, with regard to neoplastic mitoses, as an essentially negative mode of stopping, blockage, and chromial distintegration and furthermore presents a danger—without speaking of general toxicity—to the mitoses of normal cells and, among others, to that of the germinal series.

Natural Immunity

For some time already, a new orientation had been taken in the work of researchers studying cancer. As a matter of fact, the possibilities of natural immunity, as much zoological as physiological or individual in the cancer grafts, whose essentially antitissular nature remains obscure, have shown that cancer should no longer be considered a cellular disease isolated from general biological disorders. To the contrary, the evolution of this disease is linked to conditions of the organism, and the aptitude to cancerization points back to the organism "alone."

To grow, the tumor needs the organism, and without the latter cancerization cannot take place. Given the interaction that exists between the organ and the tumor, in particular its vascularization and the composition of the blood that irrigates it, as well as the state of nervous influx pertaining to it, all modification of these different factors can thus have an action on the very life of the cancer. The process that at certain times permits the host carrier of tumor to stabilize it should be analogous to that which permits an individual to harbor in his throat *diphtheria bacillis* without being stricken by this disease. It is possible that similar phenomena occur with regard to malignant cells. This is reasoning by analogy. If one considers the numerous possible causes of cancer that surround us, is it not possible that there exists in certain individuals a resistance to the development of cancer?

Grafts Studies

A number of studies have been undertaken with the purpose of clarifying this problem. The first attempts were undertaken with patients stricken with advanced cancer, who had volunteered to undergo these experiments. Some tumor fragments, removed from other persons and cultivated for a long time in an artificial medium, were implanted under the skin of their forearms. The grafts were accepted and progressively grew in volume. This result was in contradiction with the usual biological rule that requires that a tissue removed from an animal does not develop itself if it is grafted on another animal, unless the latter is a true twin of the first. The explanation of this statement, which appears to be paradoxical, requires that, with patients stricken with advanced cancer, the natural defense that opposes the acceptance of grafts had disappeared. One could inquire further if all the usual defenses of these fatigued patients had thus given up. The experiment showed that the normal defense mechanism that yielded to the cancer remained intact in all other respects. It is thus that a graft of normal tissue was rapidly eliminated. The two possible explanations were that either the cancerous tissue had a particular ability of growth contrary to the usual laws that rule grafts, or the patient had lost, especially with regard to cancerous cells, the possibilities of normal defense. The question then was: Would cancer cells transplanted to a normal individual be capable of growing?

A systematic study of this questioin had been undertaken by the cancer research center in New York, which called on volunteers from an American prison. From more than one hundred volunteers, fifty men were chosen. These men received an implant of a human cancer culture, the same type as that which had been utilized within the patients stricken with cancer. With the fifty volunteers, there had been one important defensive local inflammatory reaction, and the graft disappeared completely in four weeks. This experiment demonstrated that the human body possesses some type of resistance to the growth of cancers transplanted from another man. This resistance does not exist with patients stricken by advanced cancer. These experiments lead one to attempt to stimulate the natural defense of an organism against cancer. This is why several research projects were undertaken in the area of immunology.

It is a question of knowing if the elements that constitute the malignant tumor, essentially the chemical elements that form the cell or the nucleus, are capable of playing the role of antigen. That is to say, to provoke in the organism that contains them the formation of antagonistic substances called antibodies, whose role it is to oppose the development of the former, or antigen. If such a property can be disclosed in malignant tumors, it would indicate the possibility of promoting the formation of such antibodies for fighting against the development of cancer.

The problem is not so simple, though, because the normal tissues from which cancer results are grafted on another subject. It is necessary to suppress the antibodies thereby formed in order to verify if other antibodies exist whose formation would be due to the presence of malignant tissue. It would be necessary to admit that not the tumor but perhaps one or several elements of the cell play the role of foreign body in its development of the organism. It is possible to consider that, in certain circumstances, there exists a certain degree of antigenic properties, and that it may then be possible to promote the development and encourage the formation of corresponding antibodies. This phenomenon would then be able to explain why certain carrier subjects of cancer, although having diffused the cells from the primary tumor in the organism, do not lead to the development of other metastases. The cells stopped at other points could have provoked there the formation of antibodies that were opposed to their development or that could have destroyed them. One can equally envision a lowering of immunity that had stabilized the swarming cells, thus allowing for the development of metastases years after the destruction of the initial tumor.

Tumor Cells

The problem of cancer viewed from this angle makes it necessary to study the life of the malignant cell in order to discover which antigenic agents would be capable of producing such antibodies as are capable of destroying cancerous cells. Despite very particular aspects of the malignant cell, it is surprising to note that one may again ask how it can differ from a normal cell. Research seeking to put into evidence a new element not found in normal cells found no conclusive result. On the contrary, it would seem that there are qualitative differences in the choice made by the cell between the primary materials that supply it in particular in the chemical phenomena and the fermentations leading to the formation of nucleic acids—the role of which is essential in the life of the cell.

Tumor cells utilize more glucose than normal cells, but no quantitative differences have been found between normal tissue and tumoral tissue. This strongly indicates an increase in the formation of lactic acid. Tumor cells utilize the energy produced by the destruction of carbohydrates for the synthesis of cellular proteins at greater levels than normal cells. The cells return to a simpler form. The phenomena associated with fermentation (linked to ferments called enzymes), basic to proper life, simplify the cell, which then loses more or less those functions that individualize it and make it pertain to a specialized organ. Before the cell has utilized all its capacity for synthesis, it divides, thus prematurely interrupting the cycle of its activities and aggravating the disorder at each division. In response, it recovers former properties remembered from its origin—most important of which is the aptitude to multiply more rapidly, with consequences that are one of the manifestations of its malignancy. This abnormal growth in number is due to a liberation of the control system that normally maintains tissue harmony. The cells then become dangerous parasites or anarchists in the midst of the cellular community. The malignant cells appear "privileged and antisocial." They first monopolize materials, and, in particular, amino acids, indispensable to the life of all cells, whether normal or malignant. What is especially striking is the intensity of these physical or chemical phenomena in comparison to ordinary chemical phenomena in normal conditions. The surrounding conditions (temperature, pH, and molecular pressure) have a capital importance in the phenomena of cellular life.

Physical State of Humors

Of all the problems, the most important is, without doubt, the disorders of the humoral system engendered by these phenomena and the consequences that come from the behavior of individuals in a normal or pathological state. Hippocrates, and, well before his time, the Hebrews and the Egyptians, already attributed the major part of morbid incidents to troubled humors. By "humors," we mean the extracellular liquids of the organism. They form the fluid part of the circulating blood—the plasma—in which the sanguine elements appear, such as the suspended white and red blood cells, and also all the interstitial liquids, either lacunal or other, which bathe, impregnate, or encircle the tissue and organs. Not having a precise means of investigation, the ancients completely ignored how and why humors can be innovative. Later, when the constitution of these humors became known, medicine sought to discover which of the substances that compose these humors was responsible for the incidence of pathology. Having identified that all experimentally provoked variations, in terms of diverse humorous constitutional elements, had been powerless to reproduce the symptoms of acute or chronic disease, they came to this conclusion—diametrically opposed to that of Hippocrates: *that the humoral state plays no role in the genesis of illness.* Medicine then became "solids": Only lesions were considered important; the state of humors was left aside.

On a modern basis, we will endeavor to recognize the triumph of humoral medicine in discovering the real reason for the innovative behavior of humors, which resides not in their chemical constitution, but in the physical state of certain elements, when the latter ones change to the state of a solid. We are drawn to examine the behavior of observable elements in all biological liquids; in particular, our attention has been retained by extremely tenuous particles, whose presence has already been signaled by numerous authors at the end of the previous century.

For quite some time already, the microscope has been an indispensable instrument for precise measurement in research laboratories and the industry. The classical microscope normally permits enlargement on the order of 1800 X with a resolution of 0.1 microns. The electron microscope permits enlargement on the order of 400,000 X with a resolution of 30 to 50 angstroms. But use of the latter necessitates manipulations that alter the physical aspect of objects being observed.

We have thus perfected an instrument for microscopic observation, which we have called the *Somatoscope.* The primary quality of this apparatus is that it permits the observation of live elements and can follow the polymorphism to enlargements attaining 30,000 X with a resolution on the order of 150 angstroms. Using this instrument, we have observed, in all biological liquids and particularly in the blood, an elementary particle endowed with a movement of electronegative repulsion, possessing a polymorphic nature. We have called it the somatid. This extremely tenuous particle, whose dimension varies from a few angstroms to 0.1 microns, can be isolated and put in a culture. We could then observe the polymorphic cycle. We were surprised to discover in this cycle such elements that we had regularly seen in the blood of healthy persons but equally in the blood of carriers of diverse diseases. We made certain correlations.

In the blood of healthy persons, we observe somatids, spores, and double spores. In the course of this microcycle, we can detect the production of a *trephone*. This is a proliferative hormone indispensable to cellular division. Without it, life does not exist. In healthy individuals, the evolution of this cycle is stopped at the level of the double spore because of the presence of trephone inhibitors in the blood. These are either mineral substances, such as copper, mercury, and lead, or organic substances, such as cyanhydric acid, etc. In the course of this microcycle, the quantity of trephones necessary for cellular multiplication is thus elaborated. If, because of stress or some biological disturbances, the inhibitors in the blood diminish in concentration, the somatid cycle continues its natural evolution and one sees the appearance of diverse forms of bacteria. These have also been termed by German scientists during the 1930s *syphonospora polymorpha*.

Next come the mycobacterial forms, and then the yeast-like forms. These forms with a dimension of 4 to 5 microns evolve rapidly into ascospores, then by maturation become asci. At this stage of evolution, the ascus, after staining on a blood smear, appears as a small lymphocyte and cannot be differentiated by conventional means. Next come the filamentous forms. One can observe from an ascus the formation of a thallus in which evolves a cytoplasm of increasing importance. The cytoplasm is formed from the ascus and

a conjuncture is observable between them. It is by this conjuncture and by peristalsis that the cytoplasm forms in the
thallus. This apparent mycelial form responds to none of
the criteria of fungal elements. In fact, it is in no way affected
by massive doses of *Amphotericin B, Fungizone,* or other
antifungal agents. When this pseudomycelial element has attained its full maturity with an extremely active cytoplasm,
we then witness the bursting of this thallus and the liberation into the surroundings of an enormous quantity of new
particles capable of reinitiating a complete cycle. The empty
thallus has a fibrous aspect. Furthermore, it is often seen on
blood smears but it is considered as an artifact of the staining procedure.

From the preceding observations, we have been able to
draw the following conclusions:

1. Cellular division requires the presence of the somatid
(which is either in the animal or plant domain).

2. Trephones are elaborated by the somatid.

3. The somatid is capable of polymorphism. This polymorphism is controlled by inhibitors found in the blood.

4. A deficiency of sanguine inhibitors permits the elabo-
ration of a large quantity of trephones, which in turn lead
to disorders in cellular metabolism.

5. All degenerative diseases are a consequence of these
disorders.

In light of the above observations, the notion of "cancer,
a general disease which is localized," takes on its meaning
when one examines the evolutionary process of this affliction.
This process can be divided in two parts:

First Part: Cancerization, or initiation
When, for whatever reason, the sanguine inhibitors diminish and the polymorphism of the somatid is no longer stopped
at the double spore state, an exaggerated formation of trephones in the organism leads the cell to return to a simpler

form. The phenomena of fermentation (linked to ferments called enzymes), basic to proper life, simplifies the cell. It then loses more or less those functions that give it its individuality and make it pertain to a specialized organ. The cell is divided even before it has utilized all its capacity for synthesis, thus prematurely interrupting the cycle of its activities and aggravating its disorder at each division. In response, it recovers old properties remembered from its origin— the most important of which is the aptitude to multiply rapidly, with consequences that are one of the manifestations of its malignancy. This abnormal growth in number is due to a liberation of the control system which normally maintains cellular harmony.

At this stage, the cancerization is effective. It can be called initiation, or precancerous. We now have an accelerated and anarchic multiplication of one or several cells which provokes, by an agglomeration of their descendants, the occurrence of a new "entity" opposing the organism that had given birth to it. The immune system then enters into action and fights actively to eliminate this entity. In this fashion, we develop a small cancer daily, but our immune system rids us of it.

Second Part: Cocancerization, or promotional
If the immune system is somewhat deficient and the new entity has been able to reach a certain proportion, it then attains a "critical mass" of cells in anarchic proliferation. This entity that has been able to escape from the immune system needs an enormous quantity of nitrogen for subsistence (the cells of this entity are moreover named *nitrogen traps*). It then emits a substance that allows it to withdraw nitrogen derivatives from the organism and that, at the same time, paralyzes the immune system. We have called this substance *Cocancerogenic K Factor* (CKF).

The paralyzing action of CKF against the immune system appears only when the critical mass of cells in anarchic proliferation is reached. From this moment, the organism finds itself without defense against this new entity that can develop at will and progressively invade its host.

We can conclude from this analysis that:

1. The cancerization, or initiation, phase is linked to the reduction of sanguine inhibitors and a weakness of the immune system.

2. The cocancerization, or promotion, phase is the direct consequence of a paralyzed immune system provoked by a substance called CKF. This substance is elaborated by anarchic cells in order to withdraw, from the organism, nitrogen derivatives necessary for proliferation.

An understating of this process makes it possible to propose a therapy leading to the suppression of CKF. As a matter of fact, if the latter is neutralized, the immune system can regain its initial activity and consider each anarchic cell composing the tumors as a foreign body to be rejected.

After having carried out numerous experiments on camphor and its derivative, we have discovered that this product is endowed with remarkable pharmaceutical properties since it impedes the formation of the CKF substance, which puts leucocytes and other phagocytic elements of the organism in a state of *negative chemotaxis,* that is to say, in a state of paralysis during diverse degenerative diseases.

Camphor is neither an antimitotic nor an antimetabolite. Its property of inhibiting the CKF resides in the fact that it carries to the tumor cells all the nitrogen that it needs, suppressing by the same action the secretion that would paralyze the immune system. We have therefore proposed for experimentation a camphor derivative by the name of 714-X.

Appendix C

Gaspar Is a Miracle That Modern Medicine Can't Explain

by Ed Bantey
Reprinted from The Gazette,
Montréal, 24 December 1989

The night Gaspar came calling, I realized I hadn't held a baby in my arms for more than ten years.

Babies sense insecurity and I thought he'd howl when he found himself in my *gauche* embrace.

I mean Gaspar, who had just made his first trans-Atlantic flight, isn't just any baby.

He's the child doctors said couldn't be.

But he is, and my apprehensions proved groundless. No need even for a silly coochy-coochying. Within moments, we were friends.

Anyhow as friendly as it's possible to be with a strong, healthy boy who's yanking on one's beard.

Gaspar sized me up, gurgled a bit, and then giggled.

Perhaps it was the beard. Or the face. Or both. But I think he was happy simply to be alive.

As if he understood his mother risked her life to bring him into the world.

You may recall the Easter column about what I called Nina's "miracle" and Assurbanipal-the-Shrimp.

Now I can tell you Gaspar is the Shrimp's real name.

Like the Gaspar of the Three Wise Men who followed the star to Bethlehem for the birth of Jesus.

The moment seems appropriate for an update on our Gaspar, who also traveled a long way to see the light. He turned nine the other day. Nine months, that is.

He was born in Paris last March to Anne Vignal, the courageous Nina of the earlier column, and Renaud, her diplomat husband.

The Vignals had just arrived in Québec, where Renaud was the French consul general when Anne learned in 1984 that she had leukemia.

She was barely thirty, a superb woman with energy to burn, the classic beauty of an Old Master—and unfaltering faith.

Despite the fact doctors here, in Paris, and in New York had given her two to five years to live.

Despite the fact they said she was sterile and would never have the child she longed for.

But Anne Vignal made it against the odds. Her physical fragility was just no match for the inner strength with which she is armed—not a passive faith, but one that rejects resignation.

Anne wanted to live. And live she does.

So, while she went the only route medical science has come up with so far, she did it her way. She cut the medication dosage prescribed and turned also to alternative therapy.

Last year, when she discovered she was pregnant, the doctors were baffled and Anne was delighted.

First she called the fetus her *crevette*. Then the Shrimp became Assurbanipal. He reminded Anne of the Assyrian king who, seven hundred years before Christ, surmounted great odds to triumph over the enemy.

Finally, when the baby was born, Anne chose the name Gaspar.

Because he had made the trip to life successfully—and

because the first three letters would remind her of the man Anne credits for it all.

The man is Gaston Naessens, the sixty-five-year-old biologist recently acquitted in Sherbrooke of criminal negligence and fraud charges.

When I wrote the earlier column, I didn't identify Anne. She had told me confidentially she was using 714-X, the controversial product that landed Naessens in court.

But Renaud Vignal, now a senior official at the Quai d'Orsay, testified at the researcher's trial. So Gaspar's story is a matter of record.

Official medicine still maintains 714-X is worthless.

Frankly, I don't know if it is or it isn't. The jury was there to judge Naessens's acts, not the validity of 714-X.

Either as a *cure* for cancer or AIDS, which Naessens himself says it isn't, or as a weapon in the fight against degenerative disease, which he and some scientists say it is.

What we know is that Anne Vignal is alive, Gaspar is a thriving twenty-pounder and dozens of cancer and AIDS victims believe the product has reinforced their immune systems.

Judge Wilhelmy, who testified that 714-X helped his wife, finds it unacceptable that official medicine would deny people access to a last recourse after it has given up on them.

He's right, of course.

It's time we know if the Naessens treatment is valid.

He has offered to submit 714-X to objective analysis by qualified doctors and scientists to determine if it is effective in some cases.

It would be unconscionable to refuse that offer.

Before Naessens stands trial on further charges, Health and Welfare Canada owes it to us to oversee a detailed, case-by-case study.

Think of what it might mean to mankind if that study proved in any way positive.

Resources

As of mid-October 1990, 714-X treatment can be obtained at the Bio-Med Center (familiarly known as the "Hoxsey Clinic") in Tijuana, Baja California, Mexico. It has begun to be used experimentally on patients at the Atkins Clinic for Complementary Medicine in New York City. Other American doctors have begun to use 714-X in private practice.

Any American doctor wishing to use 714-X can send a prescription by fax to the Center for Experimental Biological Research, 5260 Rue Fontaine, Rock Forest, Québec, Canada, J1N 3B6. Instructions for use will be mailed back immediately.

714-X is presently being made available in pharmacies and to doctors in several European countries.

Index

BOOKS THAT TRANSFORM LIVES
FROM H J KRAMER INC

YOU THE HEALER:
THE WORLD-FAMOUS SILVA METHOD ON
HOW TO HEAL YOURSELF AND OTHERS
by José Silva and Robert B. Stone
*YOU THE HEALER is the complete course in
the Silva Method healing techniques presented in
a do-it-yourself forty-day format.*

WAY OF THE PEACEFUL WARRIOR
by Dan Millman
Available in book and audio cassette format
A tale of spiritual adventure . . . a worldwide best-seller!

SEVENFOLD PEACE: BODY, MIND, FAMILY,
COMMUNITY, CULTURE, ECOLOGY, GOD
by Gabriel Cousens, M.D.
*"This book expands our awareness of the dimensions of peace
so that we can all work effectively to create a world at peace."*
—JOHN ROBBINS, Author, *Diet for a New America*

An Orin/DaBen Book
OPENING TO CHANNEL:
HOW TO CONNECT WITH YOUR GUIDE
by Sanaya Roman and Duane Packer, Ph.D.
*This breakthrough book is the definitive
step-by-step guide to the art of channeling.*

An Orin/DaBen Book
CREATING MONEY
by Sanaya Roman and Duane Packer, Ph.D.
*"To be considered required reading for those who
aspire to financial well-being."*—BODY MIND SPIRIT

PURE LOVE: AFFIRMATIONS JUST FOR THIS MOMENT
by Carole Daxter
*A very special book that affirms our
connection to a safe and friendly universe.*

BIOCIRCUITS: AMAZING NEW TOOLS
FOR ENERGY HEALTH
by Leslie Patten with Terry Patten
*Biocircuits balance and magnify the body's
natural energy and are ideally suited for home use.*

TALKING WITH NATURE
by Michael J. Roads
"Reads like a synthesis of Walden *and*
The Secret Life of Plants."—EAST WEST JOURNAL

BOOKS THAT TRANSFORM LIVES
FROM H J KRAMER INC

EAT FOR HEALTH:
FAST AND SIMPLE WAYS OF ELIMINATING
DISEASES WITHOUT MEDICAL ASSISTANCE
by William Manahan, M.D.
*"Essential reading and an outstanding
selection."*—LIBRARY JOURNAL

MESSENGERS OF LIGHT:
THE ANGELS' GUIDE TO SPIRITUAL GROWTH
by Terry Lynn Taylor
*At last, a practical way to connect with the
angels and to bring heaven into your life.*

AMAZING GRAINS: CREATING VEGETARIAN
MAIN DISHES WITH WHOLE GRAINS
by Joanne Saltzman
*AMAZING GRAINS is really two books in one,
a book of recipes and a book that teaches
the creative process in cooking.*

ORIN BOOKS
by Sanaya Roman
*The Earth Life Series is a course in learning to
live with joy, sense energy, and grow spiritually.*

LIVING WITH JOY, BOOK I
*"I like this book because it describes the way I feel about
so many things."*—VIRGINIA SATIR, author, *Peoplemaking*

PERSONAL POWER THROUGH AWARENESS:
A GUIDEBOOK FOR SENSITIVE PEOPLE, BOOK II
"Every sentence contains a pearl . . ."—LILIAS FOLAN

SPIRITUAL GROWTH:
BEING YOUR HIGHER SELF, BOOK III
*Orin teaches how to reach upward to align with the
higher energies of the universe, look inward to expand
awareness, and reach outward in world service.*

JOURNEY INTO NATURE
by Michael J. Roads
*"If you only read one book this year, make that book
JOURNEY INTO NATURE."*—FRIEND'S REVIEW

JOY IN A WOOLLY COAT:
GRIEF SUPPORT FOR PET LOSS
by Julie Adams Church
*JOY IN A WOOLLY COAT is about living with,
loving, and letting go of treasured animal friends.*